Contents at a Glance

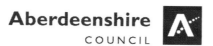

Aberdeenshire
COUNCIL

Aberdeenshire Libraries
www.aberdeenshire.gov.uk/libraries
Renewals Hotline 01224 661511

by Pat Crocker

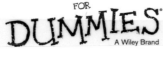

FOR
DUMMIES
A Wiley Brand

Juicing & Smoothies For Dummies®, 2nd Edition

Published by: **John Wiley & Sons, Inc.,** 111 River Street, Hoboken, NJ 07030-5774, www.wiley.com

Copyright © 2015 by John Wiley & Sons, Inc., Hoboken, New Jersey

Published simultaneously in Canada

For general information on our other products and services, please contact our Customer Care Department within the U.S. at 877-762-2974, outside the U.S. at 317-572-3993, or fax 317-572-4002. For technical support, please visit www.wiley.com/techsupport.

Wiley publishes in a variety of print and electronic formats and by print-on-demand. Some material included with standard print versions of this book may not be included in e-books or in print-on-demand. If this book refers to media such as a CD or DVD that is not included in the version you purchased, you may download this material at http://booksupport.wiley.com. For more information about Wiley products, visit www.wiley.com.

Library of Congress Control Number: 2015938130

ISBN: 978-1-119-05722-2

ISBN 978-1-119-05722-2 (pbk); ISBN 978-1-119-05718-5 (ebk); ISBN 978-1-119-05721-5 (ebk);

Manufactured in the United States of America

10 9 8 7 6 5 4 3 2 1

Table of Contents

Recipes at a Glance

Snacks

Desserts

Digestives and After Dinner

Mocktails, Cocktails, Mixers, and Punches

Exercise and Energy

Adrenal and Endocrine

Antioxidant

Detox

Elimination

Immune Boosters

Smart

Stress Reducers

Baked Goods

Soup, Sauces, and Syrups

Introduction

$\bullet$ $\bullet$

I'm excited to be updating this book, and I'm even more excited that you're reading this revised edition. I'm delighted to be sharing new science-based nutrition concepts, including all that I know about being healthy and preventing disease, along with my tips and recipes for making great smoothies and juices. In this updated version, I've added 25 new recipes that are aimed at specific healthy goals for your body. I've also updated the list of super ingredients that you can blend or whisk into smoothies and juices.

Your decision to make juices and smoothies part of your diet is truly an adventure because, although it may not give you the breathtaking adrenalin rush of bungee jumping or rock climbing, you're starting out on a journey that could change your life. You'll be doing something that may be outside your normal routine, and you'll likely be exploring options you may not have considered before. Like any good road trip, this book offers you a map — but you're the one behind the wheel. You call the shots and you determine just how much you'll benefit from this trip into health and well-being.

Do you want to lose weight? Have more energy? Get stronger? Stop getting colds? Remember more? Have vibrant skin, hair, and nails? Slow the aging process? It's all possible by eating the right foods, exercising, and including fruits and vegetables in your daily regime.

I know this because I haven't just listened to experts and read about and researched ongoing medical studies, but actually experienced the benefits of good food and a healthy diet that includes juices and smoothies. I've experienced the "juice high" from cleansing and detoxifying, and I've come to agree with dietitians, nutritionists, food scientists, and medical researchers in many fields when they say that diet, exercise, health, and well-being are inextricably entwined — modern disease is a curse that is a product of chemical pollutants; high-fat, high-sugar, highly refined and processed foods; over consumption of caffeine and alcohol; and a lack of physical exercise.

I'm thrilled that you've started on your adventure that can take you, your body, and even your mind and emotions to places you never thought you'd go. And I'm glad to be part of the spark that guides you toward drinking your way to better health.

My overall message for this second edition: Eat or drink more fruits and vegetables to be well.

About This Book

Juicing & Smoothies For Dummies, Second Edition, is a reference book. You don't have to read it straight through, from beginning to end, to get what you need out of it. Instead, you can use the table of contents and index to locate the information you need when you need it.

This new edition is loaded with juice and smoothie recipes for breakfast, lunch, dinner, and snacks as well as new recipes for healthy bodies, so you're bound to find a wide variety of drinks you'll love. If you want frozen, dessert-type recipes, go to www.dummies.com/extras/juicingandsmoothies.

But this isn't just a recipe book — I also provide a wealth of information on equipment, healthy ingredients, fruits, vegetables and herbs, and a healthy lifestyle.

Foolish Assumptions

When I wrote this book, I made a few guesses about you:

- ✔ You're interested in being healthy by increasing your intake of fruits and vegetables and by replacing one or two meals with juices or smoothies.
- ✔ You're interested in trying new juice and smoothie recipes.
- ✔ You intend to reduce or maintain a healthy weight for your height and age.
- ✔ You wish to prevent diseases, such as cancer, diabetes, and heart disease.

If part or all of this is you, you've come to the right book!

Icons Used in This Book

Icons help you to zero in on important facts and things that are worth noting. Here's a key to what the icons mean:

Anything marked with the Tip icon makes your life easier — at least when it comes to juicing and smoothies.

When I want to draw your attention to an important piece of information, I use this icon. The Remember icon indicates something I think is worth remembering.

When health or safety issues arise, the Warning icon appears. It lets you know that you need to heed with care the subject at hand.

 I don't use the Technical Stuff icon very often, but when I do, it adds some extra scientific or technical information that offers a bit more information on a topic. Feel free to ignore anything marked with this icon.

 This icon directs you to free online material that you can refer to for additional information and resources.

Beyond This Book

In addition to the content of this book, you can access some related material online. You can read a free Cheat Sheet at www.dummies.com/cheatsheet/ juicingsmoothies that contains additional information about the standards. You can also access some additional helpful bits of information at www.dummies.com/extras/juicingsmoothies, including several bonus dessert frozen smoothies.

Where to Go from Here

If you're new to juicing and smoothies, then I suggest you start with Chapters 1 and 2 to get a good feel for what you can expect.

If you're shopping for a blender or juice extractor, Chapter 3 is a good place to start. If the produce section of your local supermarket is a foreign land to you, turn to Chapter 4 for tips on shopping for fruits and vegetables. If you're not really sold on the health benefits of juicing and smoothies, check out Part II. And if all you want is to make something delicious right here, right now, turn to Parts III and IV.

Peruse the index or table of contents, find a topic that interests you, and then flip to that chapter for more information. You can then use this book as a resource guide on your juicing and smoothie journey.

I hope you achieve a healthy lifestyle that includes juices and smoothies and a whole-foods diet, because I know for a fact that it'll be a great place for you to be.

Part I
Getting Started with Juicing and Smoothies

getting started

with

Juicing & Smoothies

 web extras

To read more about the ins and outs of juicing and smoothies, refer to www.dummies.com/cheatsheet/juicingsmoothies for an online Cheat Sheet chockfull of important tips and advice.

In this part . . .

- ✔ Grasp the basics of juicing and smoothies and what they can do for you so you can incorporate them into your diet.

- ✔ Understand the type of equipment that you need to make juices and smoothies.

- ✔ Figure out your options for equipment for making juices and smoothies before you buy (don't worry, buying a juicer or blender isn't too technical).

- ✔ Refresh your shopping habits and identify the best fruits and veggies to use to make juices and smoothies.

- ✔ Know how to get the most from your fruits and veggies with tips on purchasing, cleaning, and storing them.

Chapter 1

Energizing Your Health with Juices and Smoothies

In This Chapter

▶ Looking at what juices and smoothies offer

▶ Juicing for the joy of it

▶ Savoring smoothies

*W*elcome to a healthier life through juicing and smoothies. With this book, you can regain your natural energy or life force by eating and especially by drinking to be well. Energy is the basic force throughout all of nature that drives life. It starts at the cellular level. To nourish the cells and live life at optimum health, you need four essential components: sleep, air, water, and nutrients.

You can get those nutrients from a variety of sources, but you get the most bang for your buck with whole, organic foods. Whole foods offer a wide variety of nutrients, including phytonutrients; not only are they a source of soluble and insoluble fiber, but also they're relatively low in fat. Whole, organic foods are unprocessed and unrefined, not chemically treated, and they're in as pure a state as possible when you eat them. Whole foods are fresh fruits and vegetables, whole grains, legumes, lentils, nuts, seeds, and herbs. In addition to these foods, a whole foods diet may include small amounts of unprocessed meat and dairy products.

Juices and smoothies offer immediate results and a gigantic step along the path toward health and wellness through whole foods. If you own a blender, you can start today and with very little money, time, or effort, you'll have more energy, improved digestion and elimination, a stronger immune system, a better memory, and healthy skin and nails — and you'll likely lose some weight, too.

This chapter serves as your starting point to the world of juices and smoothies. When you begin energizing your health through smoothies and juicing, you'll feel positively charged and fully able to take whatever life has to offer.

Drinking Your Energy and Health in a Glass

Opting to make your own smoothies and juices means that you're making a fresh start. Commercial juices and smoothies, whether purchased at your grocery store or at a juice bar, are still better for you than junk food and soft drinks, but making your own allows you to be in total control of what goes into the drink. You can save money and still buy organic, fresh fruits and vegetables that are at their peak of ripeness and, thus, bursting with optimum nutrients.

Reaching for a glass of homemade juice or a smoothie means that you can stop taking commercial supplements unless a doctor has prescribed these supplements. You'll save money and get more of your daily nutrient requirements by drinking two or more pure fruit or vegetable drinks every day. The advantage of consuming whole fruits and vegetables is that they contain so many complementary nutrients and trace elements, not just the major ones such as vitamin C or A. These super phytonutrients help the body metabolize or use the vitamins or minerals that you may not be able to absorb from a particular food or a commercial supplement, and they help to boost their effectiveness.

Commercial supplements that have isolated one or two nutrients lack all the other substances that occur naturally in whole foods and that allow the body to fully use them. For example, if you were taking a multivitamin with 10 mg of iron and it didn't have enough vitamin C and calcium to assist the body in taking up and using that iron, the iron would pass through your body virtually unused.

My advice for complete and optimum healthy living in a glass is to drink the rainbow twice a day. Try to include as wide a variety as possible of the vibrant and colorful fruits and vegetables available to you. This approach ensures that you're getting the best and the most nutrients that nature offers. And if you drink two or more glasses of juice or smoothies every day, you'll be providing your body with a continuous replenishment of nutrients that are lost in normal daily living. Think of your body as a bank: If you deposit only lower value coins (or empty calories), you won't have the cash (or energy) to do the things you want. Worse still, eventually, you won't have the reserves to defend yourself against a tough economy (bacteria and deadly diseases).

Eating well and adding two or more fresh juices or smoothies to your daily routine will top up your nutrient reserves all day long so that you'll actually notice a change in your energy and physical well-being. Take a peek at what you can expect from healthy living in a glass:

- **Energy to burn:** Your cells are nourished (or not) from the food you consume. By flooding your tissues with the pure nutrients that they need to function and stay healthy, you keep them strong and able to throw off minor colds and flu, which means that after a short period of time, you actually will feel energized.

- **Glowing skin:** Collagen is made up of proteins that forms the glue used by the body to connect and support tissues such as skin, bone, tendons, muscles, organs, teeth, gums, and cartilage. Vitamin C is essential in building collagen. Fruits and vegetables high in vitamin C — citrus fruit, strawberries, cabbage, and peppers — are essential for healthy skin. Vitamin A, found in apricots, carrots, spinach, and squash, protects the skin from sun damage. Skin cells are protected from aging by Vitamin E, found in dark green leafy vegetables, wheat germ, and nuts and seeds.

- **Bright eyes:** Beta-carotene, as found in the carotenoids of fruits and vegetables, is converted to retinol by the body. *Retinol* protects the surface of the eye, or the *cornea,* and is essential for good vision. Vitamin A is so important to your eyes that a deficiency (rare in developed countries) results in blindness.

- **Buff bones:** In the United States, 40 million or more people have osteoporosis or are at high risk for low bone mass, according to the National Institutes of Health. Among several other things, a diet low in calcium and vitamin D will make you more prone to bone loss. This is something you can totally control by including calcium-rich foods in smoothies and getting lots of fresh air and sunlight for vitamin D. Dark green leafy vegetables, beans, tofu, sesame seeds, and sea vegetables contain lots of usable calcium. Dairy products have calcium with vitamin D added; yogurt, milk, eggs, and cheese are good sources of vitamin D.

Jumping into Juicing

Although the water or juice of mainly fruits has been enjoyed for centuries, it wasn't until the beginning of the 20th century that two men began to look at raw juice as a medical cure. Called the *Roshåft Kur,* or raw juice cure, it was revolutionary at the time, and its developers, Dr. Max Bircher-Benner and Dr. Max Gerson, used it to promote health and well-being for patients suffering from fatigue and stress.

Just about everyone living in the 21st century suffers from fatigue and stress at some point. And raw juicing would be a quick and positive step toward repairing the damage to cells from modern-day stress.

Food flows through your gastrointestinal tract, which extends from your mouth to your bowels, and must be absorbed through the walls of the stomach and intestines before it can enter the bloodstream. Like most things associated with the body, *assimilation* (absorption of nutrients) is complicated. For total transport of nutrients through the intestinal cell wall, key enzymes and minor nutrients must be present. Once absorbed, nutrients circulate to and feed all your tissues by way of your blood. Nutrients, which are tiny molecules, are bound up in the larger cells of carbohydrate, and they're in the water or juice of fruits and vegetables. When you juice, you remove the fiber and cellulose tissue in order to leave the pure water and nutrients. In fact, by juicing, you're performing critical steps in the digestive process, which would normally start by chewing to break down the flesh of fruits and vegetables. All the nutrients in juice are instantly available for moving into the blood and, in fact, they're completely taken up and on their way to repair cells within 10 to 20 minutes of drinking them. They save the body from doing digestive work — the gallbladder, pancreas, and stomach from excreting bile and digestive enzymes and the liver from separating toxins.

A brief history of juicing

The Dead Sea Scrolls have revealed that mashing pomegranate and figs for "profound strength and subtle form" was practiced from before 150 B.C. This is perhaps the first record of man's attempt to separate the vital juices from fruits and vegetables for their healing benefits.

Throughout the ages, herbalists and other health practitioners have grated or ground fresh herbs and soft fruits and pressed the juice along with the healing, active constituents from them. Dr. Max Gerson was the first to put forth the concept that diet could be used as cancer (and other disease) therapy, but it wasn't until the 1930s, when author and raw food proponent Dr. Norman Walker invented the first juicing machine, that juicing became widely available. Cumbersome and yet effective, Walker's machine, called the Norwalk, first grates and squeezes fruits and vegetables.

The pulp is placed into a linen bag and pressed using a hydraulic press. The first of its kind and still available, the Norwalk allowed ordinary people to effectively extract the juice from fruit and vegetables.

Around the mid-1950s, the Champion machine, the first masticating juicer, was invented. The high speed (4,000 rpm) of the turning rod causes friction, which heats the juice and destroys the live enzymes and other nutrients.

In 1993, the world's first twin-gear juice extractor, called the Greenpower juicer, was produced. It's based on the old mortar-and-pestle method of pressing out the maximum living nutrients from fruits and vegetables without losing them to heat.

Today, many great makes and models of juicing machines are available.

Juices are the fastest and easiest way for the body to take up the nutrients it needs to feed and detoxify itself.

If you want to jump-start your adventure into health, jump into juicing. Today's juice machines are leaps ahead of the juicers of years ago. Chapter 3 fills you in on how to buy and care for equipment, but for now, trust me that juicing at home is more economical, faster, cleaner, and more convenient than ever before.

Savoring Smoothies

Smoothies are the darlings of the healthy-drink world. They taste divine; they can be as nutritious as a salad and as satisfying as a light lunch; they're so easy to make, drink, and clean up after; and they enrich the diet without adding too many calories or unwanted fat. Who wouldn't want to savor them?

Beyond the basics of fruit and fruit juice ingredients, smoothies are exciting in their range of possibilities and are limited only by your imagination. Although fruit smoothies are the most popular by far, vegetable smoothies can be just as rewarding, and adding milk or organic soy boosts protein and calcium.

Smoothies are a delicious, guilt-free alternative to high-sugar, high-calorie iced drinks. For people who love iced-coffee drinks, milkshakes, and the like, smoothies make the transition to healthier drinks easy. You don't need to feel deprived, and you don't have to sacrifice taste and texture while enjoying maximum health benefits. Make antioxidant iced smoothies with frozen berries, bananas or other fruit, and iced drinks (see Chapter 19) and save money while actually doing something healthy for your body.

With dairy ingredients, nuts and seeds, legumes, herbs, and protein supplements, smoothies can be used as the occasional meal replacement (see the breakfast, snack, lunch, and dinner smoothies in Chapters 16 and 17). Check out the incredible ingredients that you can add to smoothies in Chapter 15.

Here are a couple of the benefits you can enjoy by using herbs in smoothies:

- ✔ **Enhanced energy:** The American Cancer Society acknowledges that ginseng is used to provide energy, among other things. One teaspoon of powdered ginseng in smoothies no more than twice a day is all you need.

- ✔ **Improved memory:** Ginkgo biloba increases blood flow to the brain and is widely used in Europe for treating dementia; through studies, the University of Maryland Medical Center reports that ginkgo positively effects memory and thinking in people with Alzheimer's or vascular dementia. You can add drops of the tincture or stir a teaspoon of the powdered ginkgo into smoothies.

A brief history of smoothies

Around the turn of the 20th century, soda fountain jerks were hand-tossing stainless steel cups of creamy milkshakes from milk, ice cream, and flavored syrups. But the fruit smoothie hadn't even been thought of yet, nor was it possible until Fred Waring marketed Steve Poplawski's new invention, which came to be known as a *blender*.

The blender was first sold to drugstores with soda fountains and to bars and restaurants with bars. Milkshakes were the first drinks to be made in the new blender machines. These new machines didn't come to be used on the beaches of California until around the mid-1960s. The earliest fruit smoothies were thick, frozen drinks made from orange juice, strawberries, and ice, and although they shared the electric blender in common with the longer-standing milkshake, smoothies were a completely different drink aimed at cooling and refreshing beach-goers. Catering to the resurgence of macrobiotic vegetarianism in the United States, restaurants added smoothies to their menus, and the drink spread around the country.

Many commercial products have evolved since the late 1960s, and now the word *smoothie* is generic, meaning a thick drink blended from fruit juice and fruit. Today the international smoothie industry is a multibillion-dollar revenue generator with new drinks sporting supplements and herbal tinctures along with other healing substances.

Cookbook authors (like me) have expanded the smoothie category to include vegetables and dairy, bringing it right back to the milkshake. But the true smoothie will always be the icy cold fruit juice, fresh fruit, and ice beach quencher.

I like to savor fruit smoothies made from fresh local fruit in the morning. I've found that if I add ¼ cup of low-fat cottage cheese or yogurt, it gives me the protein I need for staying focused right up until about an hour before lunch. That's when I make a vegetable juice as a sort of appetizer, which keeps me sated and allows me to make really good choices about the lunch I'll have. In this way, I've found a rhythm to getting the most out of juices and smoothies.

Chapter 2

Knowing What Juices and Smoothies Are and How They Can Benefit You

In This Chapter

▶ Defining juices and smoothies

▶ Understanding the value of juices and smoothies

▶ Anticipating what juices and smoothies can do for you

Not only are smoothies and juices good for you, but they're also fun, easy, and convenient, and they taste like an indulgent treat. They make enjoying your local abundance of fresh fruits and vegetables an everyday pleasure simply by drinking them. They do so much for your body, and developing this one healthy habit is as important as deciding to quit smoking.

Reaching for fresh homemade juices or smoothies every day could be the single most important decision of your life. Why? Because it will impact your mental, physical, and emotional well-being. It will bring about even more changes in your life and in ways that you can't begin to know when you start.

The quality of your life is only as good as the quality of the foods that sustain your body. The surest way to attain the goals of health, energy, and freedom from disease is to eat a diet rich in whole foods, such as whole grains, legumes, fruits, vegetables, herbs, nuts, and seeds. Fresh smoothies and juices are bursting with proteins, carbohydrates, essential fatty acids, vitamins, minerals, live enzymes, and phytonutrients that are vital to your health.

In this chapter, I give you a close look at what makes a smoothie different from a juice. If you're wondering exactly what they do for your body, you've come to the right place — this chapter highlights the benefits of both. Finally, it helps you decide whether one or the other (or both) fits you and your lifestyle.

Defining Juices and Smoothies

Both juices and smoothies are incredibly good for your body, taste great, and can be enjoyed any time. But if you think that smoothies and juices are the same, you don't know how these healthy drinks are made and what ingredients are used to make them. In this section, I fill you in.

Juices and smoothies are made mostly of fruit and vegetables, so you may be interested to know the components that make up these foods. Whole fruits and vegetables are made up of between 80 percent and 95 percent water (this is what makes them so refreshing); the other 5 percent to 20 percent is carbohydrate or fibrous cells and nutrients (see Chapter 6).

Recognizing what juices are

Juice is the water and most of the nutrients that have been separated from much of the carbohydrate or fibrous pulp in fruits and vegetables. Sometimes a very limited number of healthy ingredients are added to juice to boost the nutritional punch, but they aren't essential (see Chapter 11).

You can squeeze or press citrus fruit (like oranges, grapefruits, and lemons) in order to get the juice, but the only way to juice other fruits and vegetables at home is to process raw, fresh fruits and vegetables through a juicing machine that presses or cuts and spins them so that the juice is extracted from the pulp.

You need a juice machine to make fresh homemade fruit or vegetable juice, and you need a citrus press to make citrus juices. You can't make juice in the blender.

Knowing what smoothies are

If I can drink the liquid that comes out of my blender, why isn't it called juice? Because the whole fruit or vegetable has been chopped so fine you may think that it's juice but because the pulp (or fiber) is still in the liquid, it isn't a juice. (Refer to the earlier section for more about what juices are.)

When a liquid (such as fresh juice, milk, or broth) and fresh fruits and/or fresh vegetables are combined in a blender and processed into a purée, the resulting drink is called a *smoothie*. The whole fruits and vegetables with the skin (if organic), but not inedible seeds, are blended until the cells in the fruit and other ingredients are so small that they're transformed into a drinkable liquid. Smoothies may have lots of other ingredients added (see Chapter 15), but the main ingredients are the liquid and the fruits and/or vegetables.

Although you may start out making smoothies with a regular kitchen blender, the best machine for all kinds of smoothies (including those that feature nuts, ice, frozen fruit or vegetables, and grains) is a high-powered, heavy-duty machine (see Chapter 3 for a comparison of several excellent brands). You can use a food processor, but the drink won't be as thick and smooth, and it may leave a mess when the bowl is removed from the base.

Differentiating between juices and smoothies

The differences in these healthy drinks are in the ingredients and the equipment used to make them. Juices are made from fresh fruits and vegetables, and that's it. You need a juicing machine to separate the juice from the pulp of the fruit or vegetable. Juices are the pure water and nutrients, including the pigments of the fruits and vegetables they're made from, so they're thin and range in color from bright green to yellow to orange to red and pink and even blue.

Smoothies, on the other hand, are made from a large range of many more ingredients. They, too, are made from fresh fruits and/or vegetables, but they have some liquid (fruit or vegetable juice, broth, milk, or yogurt) added and may include nuts, seeds, ice cream, frozen fruits or vegetables, supplements, and other health products. Smoothies are smooth and thick and tend to be lighter or more muted in color than their juice counterparts.

Introducing Juicing

With science backing the concept that diet has a direct effect on health, more and more people are coming to realize that fresh juice can be used to help prevent disease and all sorts of modern ailments. It didn't take long for gyms, clinics, health clubs, pharmacies, health or whole-food shops, homeopathic establishments, and even chain fashion stores and, of course, malls to realize that the health drink trend was something they could capitalize on.

Although you can buy commercial juices in stores and restaurants, it's still healthier, not to mention less expensive, to juice at home using fresh, organic fruits and vegetables. A whole new generation of affordable, masticating and centrifugal juicing machines that are smaller and easier to clean have made the juicing revolution a fact of modern life.

If you don't have a juicer, flip to Chapter 3 — it defines the types of juicers available and gives you great tips on what to look for in buying one. You can't make juice without a juicer.

Identifying the benefits of juicing

Juicing has many, almost too many, benefits to list. And you may find, as I did, that some benefits you just can't know until you experience them. If you get into the habit of making and consuming fresh juices twice a day, you'll sense the juice instantly release nourishment into your bloodstream. It's a close-your-eyes-and-savor-the-experience kind of moment when you tip the glass and let the brilliant liquid slide effortlessly down your throat. Taking a juice break is like a visit to a spa — relax and enjoy doing something special for yourself.

Contributing to your daily intake of fruits and vegetables

Many health professionals and institutions tell you how many fruits and vegetables to eat in a day, and as long as their minimum numbers are no less than five, they aren't exactly wrong. It's just that, in their desire to get you to eat more than the average two vegetable servings most Americans eat in a day, they're happy just to see you increase that less-than-adequate number.

What they may not explain is that if you eat at least seven and closer to ten servings of fruits and vegetables daily, the antioxidants and other phytonutrients will help reduce the risk of modern diseases such as cancer, obesity, heart disease, stroke, arthritis, asthma, macular degeneration, and diverticulosis. But man, that's a lot of fresh fruits and vegetables!

That's where juicing comes in. A single glass of juice may consist of one apple, two carrots, one beet, a piece of ginger, and half a lemon. It delivers a full serving of fruit, along with three servings of vegetables — all in one drink.

You can dramatically increase your daily intake of fruits and vegetables by drinking smoothies and juices.

Preventing modern diseases

People don't get scurvy nowadays, but from as far back as Hippocrates in 400 B.C., it was a dreaded and fatal disease. Long-voyage sailors ate fresh lemons or limes to prevent scurvy (hence the nickname "limeys" for Englishmen). Jacques Cartier, a 16th-century North American explorer relied on native people, who gave him a boiled tea of juniper needles and saved them when they had tried to overwinter in what is now Nova Scotia. The action of preventing scurvy was called *antiscorbic* long before anyone knew about vitamin C.

The discovery of vitamin C around the turn of the 20th century was a major turning point for food research. People have come a long way in understanding just what's in the foods they eat. Today they know the science behind what the ancients knew from experience — that fruits and vegetables actually prevent diseases. They also know that they need to eat a wide variety to ensure that they get the full spectrum of offered nutrients. Here's a quick highlight of what juices and smoothies have to offer (see Chapters 7 and 8 for more):

- ✔ **Fiber:** Only fruits and vegetables contain soluble and insoluble fiber, which controls blood glucose levels to prevent diabetes, reduces cholesterol and the risk of heart disease, and reduces the risk of diverticulosis and a variety of cancers.

- ✔ **Antioxidants:** Found mostly in fruits and vegetables (along with red wine and dark chocolate), antioxidants reduce the risk of coronary heart disease, reduce cell damage, and prevent aging and cancers.

- ✔ **Phytonutrients:** The phytonutrients in fruits and vegetables prevent a variety of human ailments, including arthritis, diabetes, and osteoporosis.

- ✔ **Vitamins and minerals:** More than any other foods, fruits and vegetables are high in these essential nutrients that build and repair cells and tissue, protect against colds and flu, and keep the organs and glands functioning at their best.

Phytonutrients and trace elements are like keys opening the door for vitamins and minerals to be taken up by the body. They're missing from manufactured supplements, so the body misses out on all the benefits from the vitamin or mineral you thought it was getting. (See the nearby sidebar, "The synergistic value of complete nutrients" for more.)

Building a stronger immune system

Immunology (the study of the immune system) is a growing and dynamic field. The immune system includes the lymphatic organs (thymus, spleen, tonsils, and lymph nodes) and white blood cells, along with other specialized cells. Its prime function is to protect the body against infection and diseases.

Factors that cripple the immune system are stress, free radicals, nutritional deficiencies, sugar, obesity, fats in the blood, and alcohol. So it makes sense to eliminate those factors from your life.

The synergistic value of complete nutrients

Juices and smoothies are made from whole fruits and vegetables, so they contain all the particular nutrients found in those foods — including other vitamins and minerals, enzymes, trace elements, phytonutrients, and even some active components that haven't yet been discovered. Commercial supplements isolate one or two major nutrients like the B complex of vitamins or calcium, and they fail to include all the more subtle phytonutrients that make it easy for the body to assimilate and use the larger ones.

Foods are synergistic. The interaction of the nutrients found in fruits and vegetables, as well as all whole natural foods, has a sum total benefit that outweighs the benefit of each food's individual nutrients. That's why you can't isolate just one vitamin or mineral in a supplement for optimum nutrition. Eating the whole fruit or vegetable is synergistic, meaning that those foods work together to provide the optimal level of vitamins and other nutrients for optimum health.

Quite simply, natural whole foods and the nutrients found in them are best adapted to the human digestive system. The body knows what to use and what to discard. Only by consuming the whole fruit or vegetable can you be sure that the vitamins and minerals you know are in those foods will be taken up by the bloodstream and used by your cells.

The American Cancer Society agrees that a diet rich in fruit, vegetables, beans, and grains is more beneficial than taking phytochemical supplements.

You've taken the first step in building a stronger immune system by becoming interested in your health. Optimal immune function requires a healthy diet (including juices), exercise, and a positive mental attitude.

Improving memory

Memory and cognition problems can be a result of many things, including poor nutrition and amino acid balance, allergies, *candidiasis* (yeast infection), thyroid disorders, low blood sugar, and poor circulation to the brain. However, a general decline in mental performance is caused most often by free radical damage. Juicing with fruits and vegetables that are high in antioxidants (see Chapter 20) protects all the body's cells, including the brain, from the ravishing effects of the unstable oxidizing free radicals.

Table 2-1 lists some brain-boosting nutrients that you can get from fresh, organic juices.

Understanding raw, live enzymes, and phytonutrients

Phytochemicals are simply chemicals extracted from plants (*phyto* meaning from plants). They include nutrients that are called *antioxidants, flavones, isoflavones, catechins, anthocyanins, isothiocyanates, carotenoids, allyl sulfides,* and *polyphenols,* among others.

Only a small number have actually been discovered, named, and studied, and that's the main reason why nutritionists urge us to eat a wide variety of whole natural foods, including fruits and vegetables. In Chapter 5, you find a list of some of the most widely studied phytonutrients and an explanation of what they do for the body.

Although they have many benefits, perhaps the most important function of phytochemicals is that some of them help prevent the formation of *carcinogens* (substances that cause cancer); they block the action of carcinogens or they act on cells to suppress cancer development.

Many experts, including the American Cancer Society, suggest that people can reduce their risk of cancer significantly by eating more fruits, vegetables, and other foods from plants that contain phytochemicals.

One of the main reasons why raw food proponents claim the advantages of fresh juice and natural, uncooked whole foods is that they contain "live" active enzymes. Enzymes are minutest components of plant foods that work with vitamins and other nutrients to facilitate digestion through chemical reactions in the body. Heating by cooking and pasteurization kills enzymes, so by drinking raw fresh juice, the enzymes in the juice actually save the body from using its own enzymes. This allows energy to be shifted from digestion to other body functions like cell repair, protection, and rejuvenation.

Table 2-1	Brain-Boosting Nutrients	
Nutrient	**Function**	**Which Juice Ingredients Have It**
Choline	Essential for brain development in fetuses and infants; helps prevent memory loss associated with aging; protects the liver from damage	Lecithin, peppers, green beans, cabbage, spinach, seaweed, spirulina, cauliflower, almonds, and navy beans
Vitamin C	Boosts brainpower	Cabbage, peppers, kale, parsley, broccoli, cauliflower, strawberries, papayas, and mangoes

(continued)

Table 2-1 *(continued)*

Nutrient	Function	Which Juice Ingredients Have It
Boron	Sharpens short-term memory and attention; improves performance on mental tasks; protects against aging	A wide range of fruits and vegetables, including avocadoes, beans, carrots, pears, bananas, almonds, and walnuts (finely chopped)
Glutathione	Increases the flow of blood and oxygen to the brain; has a protective effect on brain cells; boosts mental functions	Asparagus, citrus fruit, watermelon, cauliflower, tomatoes, strawberries, and broccoli

Increasing energy

The process of digestion, something most people never think about, can be so complex and take so much energy. Digestion involves chewing and grinding food, as well as chemical processes that require enzymes to release small nutrients into your system to break food into smaller molecules. Proteins, carbohydrates, and fats all require a different set of enzymes to unlock their key components. And the whole process takes energy.

When you present your digestive system with pure raw fruit or vegetable juice, there is no digestive process that has to take place because the nutrients in the water have already been extracted from the carbohydrate and fiber. So you give your digestive system a break and allow the energy that would have gone into breaking down the food go to repairing and protecting cells.

Improving sex drive

Hormones hold the key to sexual desire or the ability to function sexually. A healthy, high-fiber, low-fat diet; exercise; and freedom from stress, especially psychological issues, all can contribute to sexual vitality. Raw foods, especially vegetables, contribute to hormone health and healthy libido.

Both vitamin C and zinc have been shown to assist in the production of testosterone and sperm. The best Vitamin C juice sources are cabbage, strawberries, spinach, citrus fruit, broccoli, kale, and peppers. The best zinc juice sources are ginger, turnips, parsley, carrots, garlic, spinach, cabbage, and grapes.

Improving digestion and elimination

As people age, their stomachs produce less acid, and breaking down food becomes a problem — it seems to occur between the ages of 35 and 45. If the body isn't digesting food properly, the nutrients don't enter the bloodstream, and all sorts of deficiencies can occur, even if you're eating normally.

Drinking raw fruit and vegetable juices gives your body a break by delivering ready-to-use nutrients. There are also some excellent digestive enzymes found in some fruits, vegetables, and herbs including pineapple, papayas, fennel, ginger, and licorice. (See Chapters 12 and 13 for digestive juice recipes.)

Fiber is the one key factor in the body's ability to eliminate waste on a regular basis. Include sources of both soluble and insoluble fiber in your diet by opting for plant foods, smoothies, and vegetable juices.

Losing weight

Because it impacts heart disease, stroke, and diabetes, *obesity* (defined as being 20 percent over the recommended weight) is considered to be a leading cause of heart disease, cancer, and ultimately, death in the United States.

Juice from fresh fruits and vegetables is virtually fat-free, and juice from vegetables is low in sugar. Drink them on a regular basis, and two things happen: You start to lose your appetite for high-fat, high-calorie junk foods, and you start to feel better, with more energy to get up and get active. See Chapter 6 for more information on how juices and smoothies can set you on a healthy diet for losing weight and increasing health.

Juicing can be the spark that helps you burn more calories than you take in.

Getting clearer skin and healthier nails and hair

Nutritional deficiencies show up first in your hair, nails, and skin, and juicing is the best way to address low levels of nutrients at the cellular level. Here are some vital nutrients for clear skin and healthy nails and hair:

- ✔ **Vitamin C:** Fruits and vegetables that are high in vitamin C — such as cabbage, strawberries, tomatoes, citrus fruit, and peppers — help to build collagen, which gives firmness as well as elasticity to skin to prevent wrinkles and leathery texture; neutralize free radicals to help reduce aging effects; and promote glowing skin, nails, and hair.

- ✔ **Vitamin A:** Vitamin A protects the skin from sun damage that leads to skin cancer, balances skin oils, provides a healthy skin color, and assists in treating blemishes. It's important for the health of the root and bulb of the hair follicles. Deficiency results in dry, brittle nails. Apricots, mangoes, cantaloupe, carrots, spinach, kale, sweet potatoes, parsley, collard greens, turnip greens, and squash are high in vitamin A.

✔ **Vitamin E:** Vitamin E is found in dark green leafy vegetables, wheat germ, nuts, and seeds. It protects skin cells from aging.

✔ **B-complex vitamins:** The B vitamins are responsible for preventing hair loss and graying hair. A deficiency of B vitamins causes fragile nails. The best juice source of B vitamins is leafy green vegetables. Whole, unrefined grains; poultry; fish; eggs; nuts; beans; and meats are food sources.

✔ **Biotin:** Deficiency contributes to hair loss. The best food sources are brewer's yeast, soy products, brown rice, eggs, walnuts, pecans, barley, oatmeal, and sardines.

✔ **Iron:** Low levels of iron in tissues can cause hair loss and fragile, brittle, ridged, or thin nails. The best juices sources are parsley, beet greens, chard, dandelion greens, broccoli, cauliflower, strawberries, asparagus, blackberries, cabbage, cucumbers, and alfalfa.

Why homemade beats bottled any day

It's no secret that many commercial juices contain high amounts of sugar and salt, but did you know that most juices are extracted using chemical methods? Orange juice, for example, is available in two forms: frozen concentrated and not-from-concentrate (which is perceived as being better because it hasn't been reduced and then re-constituted with filtered water). But the fact is that both the concentrated and the "100 percent fresh-picked oranges, nothing added, nothing taken away" juice is a heavily processed product that has been *de-oxygenated* (stripped of oxygen) in order for it to sit in vats for up to a year before it's packaged, distributed, sold in stores, and consumed. All heat-sensitive nutrients and live enzymes are gone from this juice before it ever hits your fridge. In fact, if flavor and fragrance weren't added to these juices, they "would taste like sugar water," according to Alissa Hamilton, author of *Squeezed: What You Don't Know About Orange Juice.*

Even if commercial juice were high-quality and still had its nutrients, the packaging process can be deadly because the acid from juice in cans leeches metal from the can; wax and chemicals used to make cartons contaminate juice packed in them; and shrink-wrapped cartons of juice have been exposed to high heat in the shrink-wrap process.

To be fair, there are small, independent juice producers that don't use filtered water and attempt to provide high-quality juice. These juices are packaged in glass bottles and they're thicker and cloudier, with some sediment because more of the whole fruit has been used to make them.

Bottom line: Nothing beats fresh juice from fresh, organic produce taken right after juicing.

Fresh juice versus eating the whole fruit or vegetable

As important as fresh juice is, it can't totally replace whole fruits and vegetables in your diet. The fiber in fruits and vegetables is vitally important to your health, and that essential component is removed with the carbohydrate pulp when you juice.

Having said that, juice is still extremely important in delivering the full range of nutrients that fruits and vegetables have to offer. Juice is easier for your body to digest precisely because it doesn't contain fiber or starch and added sugars. This makes it an excellent drink for snacks and for cleansing or detoxing.

Smoothies are made by chopping up the whole fruit or vegetable in order to make them drinkable. This means that you're drinking the pulp and fiber along with the pure water and nutrients — exactly as though you were eating the whole fruit or vegetable.

Bottom line: Drinking two or three vegetable juices and one smoothie and eating whole foods including mostly plants (whole grains, fresh fruits and vegetables, beans and legumes, herbs, and nuts and seeds) is the best possible day-to-day diet for optimum health.

The Lowdown on Smoothies

Smoothies are thick, they taste delicious, they usually satisfy longer than juices, and best of all, they're a delicious way to deliver whole fruits and vegetables to your body. Smoothies make a considerable contribution to your daily consumption of fiber, fruits, and vegetables, and because they're made in the blender, a machine that most households already have, they're fast and easy to clean up after making. This makes them good breakfast and snack choices that easily fit into the demands of work and family. If you teach your children good smoothie habits and have fresh fruits, vegetables, and other smoothie ingredients on hand, as older children and teens, they'll be making their own incredibly healthy after-school snacks.

Small, single-serving blending machines can make smoothie lunches or midday snacks even more appealing to working people. It's just so darn easy to savor the fresh fruit and vegetable drinks as alternatives to any junk-food snack or fast-food meal. Smoothies can play a vital role in a weight-loss program because, unlike juices that exclude the pulp, the fiber in smoothies helps stave off hunger.

For people who want to be sociable without drinking alcohol, fresh and frozen smoothies offer exciting, sophisticated alternatives at social gatherings.

The recipes in this book include a wide range of sweet and savory smoothies that will kick-start your day, maximize nutrients and supplements, and revitalize your body's digestive system. They run the gamut from breakfast, lunch, and dinner; dessert and cocktail/mocktail smoothies; to frozen and iced granitas and sherbets. See Chapters 16 to 19 for flavor and ingredient combinations for smoothies that are refreshing and luscious delights.

Examining the benefits of smoothies

Like their healthy juice counterparts, smoothies may be made from a wide array of organic, fresh fruits and vegetables. But smoothies are different from juices in two important ways: First, they're made from the whole fruit or vegetable, so they keep the pure water, nutrients, and the fiber. Secondly, so many more natural and healthy ingredients like oats, nuts, seeds, herbs, and other natural supplements may be blended with smoothies.

They're a good source of fiber

Fiber is the indigestible substance found only in plant foods, fruits, vegetables, grains, and legumes. Eating fiber is one of the easiest and least expensive ways to prevent disease and maintain health because it helps the body to eliminate waste materials and deadly toxins.

Water-soluble fiber lowers cholesterol and stabilizes blood sugar. Insoluble fiber increases stool bulk and promotes bowel movement, scouring the intestinal walls of toxic waste matter, promoting colon health by reducing the risk of diverticulosis and colon cancer.

Because they're liquidized or finely chopped whole fruits and vegetables, smoothies contain both soluble and insoluble fiber from those plants. For an even extra fiber boost, add psyllium, nuts, seeds, cooked beans or lentils, bran, and oats to smoothies.

High-fiber fruits and vegetables include apples, oranges, berries, pears, figs, prunes, broccoli, cauliflower, Brussels sprouts, and carrots.

They're a healthy substitute for empty-calorie drinks

It's precisely because smoothies contain fiber and other slow-digesting ingredients like nuts, seeds, yogurt, coconut oil, milk, or tofu that they stay with you longer and satisfy you so much more than coffee or soda.

Smoothie bars: Choosing the right blend

You think you're making a healthy choice by slurping up that healthy-sounding, creamy drink from a fast-food outlet or popular smoothie bar. If the drink has low-fat milk or fresh juice, fresh fruit, and ice, you can likely go ahead and enjoy. But if it's made from ice cream, powdered cream, sugars (glucose, fructose, corn syrup, or molasses), or any other of the high-calorie ingredients, you may be in for a shock at the calories and chemicals that are lurking in that iced refresher.

On average, depending on the outlet, 16 ounces of a commercial smoothie drink contains 260 to 320 calories. If you know the ingredients are fresh and not processed and if you're replacing a dinner with a high-protein smoothie, the higher calories may not impact your daily intake in a negative way. The point is to know exactly what goes into your drink and how to make it work as part of your daily calorie intake.

It's true that you can add all sorts of high-calorie or high-fat ingredients to homemade smoothies, but you're still in control of the quality of the organic fruits and vegetables (as opposed to it being a frozen pulp with additives); you can opt for low-fat dairy ingredients; and you can be sure that the juice is fresh, not containing filtered water or extra sweeteners.

Bottom line: Homemade smoothies beat out commercial blends hands down.

My own health routine is to have a fruit smoothie made with skim milk, 1 cup of fresh or frozen berries, an orange, half a banana, and ¼ cup of yogurt, cottage cheese, or tofu in the morning before work. This is enough to keep me feeling satisfied until lunch at noon. Sometimes I have the same drink at midafternoon to keep my blood sugar levels even and to prevent me from feeling like I'm starving, although a vegetable juice is usually enough to keep me satisfied until dinner.

They make an excellent meal replacement

Busy times call for smart choices instead of fast foods. Smoothies are smart meal replacements because they're high in nutrients. If you add small amounts of protein and even some grain to a vegetable smoothie, you can build that drink into a powerful meal replacement.

Excluding all your meals and taking only juices and smoothies isn't wise, because, as nutritionists always point out, people need a wide variety of whole, natural foods. Excluding the other plant foods like whole grains, beans, legumes, nuts, and seeds means that you're limiting the nutrients your body receives.

Breakfast and lunch are the best meals to use smoothies as a replacement for, especially if you usually skip breakfast and find yourself grabbing a fast meal for lunch. Check out Chapters 17 and 18 for great lunch and dinner smoothie recipes.

They're an easy way to take medicines, herbs, or supplements

Often the elderly or people recovering from surgery can handle smoothies long before they can tolerate solid foods. You can blend prescribed medications (only those that are meant to be taken with food) right into the smoothie, making them a nourishing drink for recovering patients. You also can boost the caloric content of smoothies by adding omega-3 rich oils, using whole milk, and adding protein sources. This is often the best way to bolster the diets of elderly and undernourished patients.

Healing herbs, tinctures, and teas can be used as smoothie ingredients. Healthy supplements like lecithin, bee pollen, goji berries, whey protein powder, activated almond butter, and green sprouts may be added to the blender along with the ingredients.

How to drink juices and smoothies year-round

I can just see you thinking to yourself, "Okay, but if I'm supposed to buy only in-season fruits and vegetables, how can I drink my favorite juices and smoothies year-round?" Fear not — here are some tips:

✔ **Buy in bulk and freeze the extra when local produce is in season.** You don't need to thaw it if you're making smoothies, and you only need to partially thaw it if you're juicing. (See www.dummies.com/extras/juicingsmoothies for ways to freeze them in the future.)

✔ **Look for organic, local frozen summer fruit, sometimes found in local whole/health stores.** If that isn't available, buy organic imported and use it in smaller amounts with fresh or frozen local fruit.

✔ **Buy organic canned fruit when those fruits are out of season.** Look for and buy fruit packed in water or light syrup because you won't want the extra calories from added sugar. If you use canned fruit packed in water, you can add the liquid to the juice or smoothie and you won't be pouring out the water-soluble vitamins.

Chapter 3

Gearing Up for Healthy Drinks

In This Chapter

▶ Choosing a juicer that's right for you

▶ Knowing what to look for in a blender

▶ Maintaining your machines to get the most from them

*N*ot until the 1930s did the perfection of the small electric motor lead to the invention of juicers and blenders. At first, only restaurants and other industrial establishments used these machines. The practice of using a juicer or blender in the home kitchen hasn't been around for much more than three generations.

Many people now own or are familiar with using a blender, and juice machines are quickly becoming essential in home kitchens as well. If you've decided that juicing is important to your health and you want to include juicing in a health regimen, this chapter is worth reading because it explains everything you need to know about the kinds of machines available today and what features to look for when buying a juicer.

If you're in the market for a blender, this chapter doesn't leave you empty-handed. I've personally tested several high-performance brands in order to show you how each one stacks up, and I give you the tips you need to find the right one for you. I also share how to care for and maintain your juicer and blender, so they'll serve up delicious, healthy drinks for years to come.

Choosing a Juicer

If you want to buy a juicing machine, this is the place to start. In this section, I explain the three main types of juicers and help you decide which one is right for you.

Eyeing the types of juicers

Knowing your level of engagement in the process of juicing is critical to matching the type of juicers available to your lifestyle, your health needs, and your expectations about convenience, so ask yourself the following questions and keep your answers in mind as you read about the types of machines available and their advantages or disadvantages.

- ✔ How much time do I want to spend making juice?

- ✔ Will my juice be a once-a-day quick snack or a health ritual that I want to put time and effort into?

- ✔ Am I fanatical about extracting the most juice from my fruits and vegetables and obtaining the highest quality nutrients, or does convenience trump any slight increase in nutrients?

 You can get the scoop on fresh raw juices by dropping in on a juice bar in a whole-food or health food store, gym, or spa. Try a fresh juice and see if you even like the taste (although that isn't usually an issue — juices are so good!). You also can see firsthand how the machine works and talk to someone who knows about the types of machines available.

Centrifugal force juicers

This type of juicer takes fruits and vegetables through a feed tube and directly into contact with a blade that shreds them. The juice from the fruits and vegetables is thrown by centrifugal force of the spinning basket toward the sides of the basket and pushed through it into a jug (or glass). If you have a continuously ejecting juicer, the pulp is forced out of the machine and into a pulp container. If the pulp isn't automatically removed from the spinning basket, the basket becomes full and you have to stop the machine, remove the pulp, and empty the basket before continuing to juice.

Here are the advantages of centrifugal force juicers:

- ✔ They have the fewest number of parts of all the juicers, which makes them fast and easy to assemble and clean.

- ✔ They're the fastest at extracting juice from fruits and vegetables, especially if the feed tube is wide enough to take a whole apple, cucumber, or orange and if the pulp is automatically ejected.

- ✔ They handle soft fruits better than the masticating juicers.

- ✔ They're the most popular types of juicers, so you have many brands with different features from which to choose.

- ✔ They stand upright and take up less space on the counter.

Although some brands are available for less, you should expect to pay between $200 and $300 for a high-quality centrifugal juicer. If you have more than $300 in your budget, consider a masticating juicer, which I discuss in the next section.

And here are the disadvantages of centrifugal force juicers:

- ✔ More oxidation of nutrients takes place as evidenced by the amount of foam on top of fresh juices from this type of juicer. (The nutritional quality is still excellent, especially if you drink the juice immediately and don't store it).
- ✔ In general, less juice is extracted from centrifugal juicers. (Some really good brands are available that produce a fairly dry pulp with not much juice waste.)
- ✔ Unless they have variable speeds, most of these types of juicers won't effectively process wheatgrass and other fine grasses.

Many people think that because the spinning basket causes friction and may get hot, more nutrients, especially live enzymes, are destroyed. The reality is that in order to destroy live enzymes in raw fruits and vegetables, the basket would have to reach temperatures of 118° F or more, which doesn't happen in any juicing machine.

Bottom line: These machines are for people who want to juice for the nutritional benefits but want to do it with as little effort, monetary investment, and time as possible.

Masticating juicers

Making use of a single *auger* (gear) that's spiral in shape, masticating juicers press and chew, or *masticate,* the fruits and vegetables as they're fed into the tube. Juice is slowly extracted and collected in a container that fits under the gear shaft, and the pulp is continuously ejected at the end of the gear shaft into a pulp container.

Here are the advantages of masticating juicers:

- ✔ They work at a low rpm so they extract more juice from the fruits and vegetables and excel at juicing leafy greens, wheatgrass, and other grasses.
- ✔ The slower speed preserves slightly more nutrients than are preserved by centrifugal force juicers because there is less oxidation.
- ✔ They can function as grain mills and make nut butters and baby food.
- ✔ They can process frozen fruits, such as bananas and strawberries, for instant frozen treats.

Here are the disadvantages of masticating juicers:

- Due to the softer, lower fiber content of fruit, masticating juicers aren't as efficient at juicing fruit as are centrifugal juicers. You need to include vegetables with fruit in order for the harder vegetables to help push the fruit through the screen.

- Some have more parts that must be assembled and cleaned.

- They have relatively small feed tubes in order to accommodate the size of the auger, which means that the food has to be cut into small pieces and fed one by one through the tube.

- As a result, juicing with a masticating juicer takes longer from assembly and cleaning, to preparing the fruits and vegetables to waiting as each small piece or leaf is fed through the tube and into the auger.

- Most are larger, wider machines that take up more counter space and aren't easy to move around. One exception is the Breville Juice Fountain Crush (BJS600XL) upright masticating juicer.

Bottom line: If you want the very most nutrients possible and you're willing to spend more time juicing, a masticating type juicer is the machine for you, especially if you plan to juice grasses and you don't have a high-performance blending machine to make sorbets and nut butters.

Triturating juicers

Similar to a masticating, single-gear juicer, the triturating juicer has two augers, and it separates the juice in two stages: First, it crushes fruits and vegetables; then it presses the juice out of them. This method of extracting juice releases more soluble fiber, enzymes, vitamins, and trace minerals from the pulp, making the juice extremely nutrient-rich. Some of these juicers actually have technology to slow down the oxidation process, which is important if you want to juice a day's worth of juice at one time and store for consumption later.

Here are the advantages of triturating juicers:

- Of all the types of juicers, they extract the most nutrients from fruits and vegetables.

- The twin augers of triturating juicers turn at a lower rpm than masticating juicers and extract more juice from a wide range of leafy greens, grasses, herbs, and hard and soft fruits and vegetables.

- They homogenize food to make baby foods, nut butters, fruit sorbets, and pasta.

And here are the disadvantages of triturating juicers:

- ✔ They're the most expensive of the three types of juicers.
- ✔ They're slow and have the disadvantages of masticating juicers in that the food must be cut up.
- ✔ They're large and imposing machines that take up more space on a counter.

 Bottom line: This machine is for you if you already own a juicer and want to move to the next level or if you know you're dedicated to a juicing regime and don't mind the extra cost to get the very best nutrients from leafy greens, herbs, and a wide variety of vegetables and fruits.

Wheatgrass juicers

These limited-function machines may be manual (hand-cranked) or electric. They're designed to juice wheatgrass and other grasses, herbs, sprouts, and leafy greens. They also handle very soft fruit like berries, grapes, and kiwifruit.

Here are the advantages of wheatgrass juicers:

- ✔ They're simple to use.
- ✔ They're one-purpose machines that are good at extracting juice from grass, greens, and soft fruits.
- ✔ They're relatively inexpensive.

Here are the disadvantages of wheatgrass juicers:

- ✔ They're one-purpose machines that require another purchase if you want to juice hard fruits and vegetables.
- ✔ Cheaper models have plastic blades, which are inferior (so be sure to look for machines that have stainless steel blades).

 Bottom line: Wheatgrass juicers are a good choice if you want to process only greens and soft fruits. If you want to have the option of juicing other fruits and vegetables along with wheatgrass, put the money toward either the masticating or the triturating juice machines, which can handle everything the wheatgrass juicers can, but with many more options.

Juice presses

Also called citrus presses, these juicers are designed to squeeze the juice from oranges, tangerines, grapefruit, lemons, and limes. They range from simple handheld reamers or one-handed lemon/lime presses to powerful electric presses that will juice and automatically strain dozens of orange or lemon halves one at a time but quickly and with little effort.

Manual presses

Glass, ceramic, and plastic juicers are designed to sit on top of a glass or bowl or have a reservoir large enough to hold the juice from one-half lemon or one-half orange. Ceramic lemon/lime presses squeeze the juice from one-half lemon or one-half lime while catching and straining the seeds. This type of handheld press is handy for single drinks.

Here are the advantages of manual presses:

- They're inexpensive and easy to use and clean.
- They're easy to store in a drawer.

Here are the disadvantages of manual presses:

- It's slow and tedious to juice more than two or three citrus fruits at a time.
- You have to strain out the seeds using a strainer.

Electric presses

Electric juice presses are powerful enough to press an unlimited number of citrus fruit halves, and most have a strainer built into the machine. They're easy to use and clean.

Here are the advantages of electric presses:

- You can juice dozens of citrus fruit at a time.
- The machine parts are easy to clean.

Here are the disadvantages of electric presses:

- They're more expensive than manual presses.
- They take up more space on a counter.

Features to look for in a juicer

You want to find a brand that has as many of the features you want within your budget. Here are some features to consider before you make your final purchase decision.

Simplicity: Easy to assemble and use, easy to clean

If you want to enjoy health benefits from juicing, but you aren't passionate, keeping it simple is the best route. If your juicer has only a few simple parts and is easy to use and clean, you'll be motivated to use it more often.

Keeping the juicing machine on the counter is also essential to simplicity. A sleek, upright centrifugal machine takes up the least amount of space, is incredibly fast, and is easy to assemble and clean.

If you're highly motivated or if you already own a fairly inexpensive juicer and you want to move up to a machine that juices grasses and extracts more juice and nutrients, the masticating or triturating juicers are a better choice.

Speed: High speed and variable speed

Masticating and triturating juicers have only one speed: slow and slower, respectively, which is a health advantage.

Some centrifugal juicer models come with variable speeds, which slow the blades of the spinning basket down for soft fruit and allow you to gradually increase the speed as you juice harder fruits and vegetables. The slower the basket spins, the more juice may be extracted from the fruit or vegetable, so this is a definite advantage of these types of machines.

Number and quality of nutrients extracted

Masticating or triturating juicers are generally thought to be better at extracting and preserving the nutrients. However, because you have to cut up the fruits and vegetables into very small pieces, depending on how long they sit out, they may lose nutrients to oxidation before they even hit the auger.

Efficiency

You're making an investment, and you want to be sure that a juicing machine is efficient in doing the things that you consider to be important. If possible, get a live demonstration of the juicer in action. Consider the following:

- ✔ **The amount of juice extracted:** Masticating or triturating juicers are thought to be better at extracting the juice, but my experience with a centrifugal juice machine (particularly with the Breville Juice Fountain Multi-Speed) is that the pulp is pretty dry if you use the variable speed function and don't apply any pressure to the fruit or vegetable as it passes down the feed tube.

- ✔ **External pulp ejection:** Unless you only ever plan to juice one serving at a time, this is a critical feature to any juicing machine. Masticating or triturating juicers continually expel the pulp, so this isn't an issue. Some centrifugal juice machines don't have a continual expulsion feature so you have to stop the machine in order to clean out the basket.

- ✔ **Yield of juice and dryness of pulp:** If you can see a demonstration of the machines you're interested in buying, you can measure the juice extracted from the same fruits or vegetables. Wet pulp is an indication that the machine is not effective in extracting a high yield of juice.

✔ **Size of the feed tube:** Masticating or triturating and some brands of centrifugal juicers have a very small feed tube, which means the food must be cut into small pieces or leaves must be fed one by one into the machine. If you know you want a centrifugal juicer, be sure that the model you choose has a feed tube large enough to take a whole apple, orange, or cucumber. This feature makes the preparation easy because the food doesn't require cutting and chopping. A good size for a centrifugal juicer is 3 inches or wider, whereas masticating juicers may have a wide funnel that feeds into the narrow feed tube, but you still have to cut the fruit or vegetables into smaller pieces.

✔ **Size of the pulp container:** The larger the pulp bin, the more efficient the juicer is because you don't need to stop and empty it when juicing large amounts of fruits or vegetables.

✔ **Multipurpose:** Masticating or triturating juicers are able to grind coffee beans, spices, and nuts for nut butter, and can make baby food. If you plan to use all of these functions, the extra cost may be worth it.

Reliability

Like a car or boat or any other appliance, you want to have the luxury of using a juicer for a very long time in order to get the most from your investment. Consider the following:

✔ **Quality of the parts:** The quality of the parts and the materials used are one indication of reliability. Stainless steel outperforms and outlasts plastic and is easier to clean. The other determining factor in assessing reliability is the size of the motor.

✔ **Motor size:** It takes a considerable amount of power to rip through tough fibers of vegetables like beets and turnips, and a juicer with insufficient power will slow down or even burn out over time, so look for a juicer with the most powerful motor in your price range. A reliable motor size is 1.1 horsepower (Hp) or higher.

Noise

Some juice machines are extremely loud during use. Noise is a huge issue to some people, especially if they live with people who might be sleeping when they want to juice.

Warranty

Although most high-end juicers come with a seven-year motor warranty, some brands offer a ten-year or even 15-year motor warranty, which indicates the manufacturer's confidence in the durability of the motor.

Choosing a Blender

Blenders remain a popular kitchen tool, and with the exception of touch pad and computer technology, their basic design has changed little in the 80 years they've been in existence. They're very good at what they do, and the only machine to ever come close to eclipsing their use is the food processor. Still, for puréeing foods and blending liquid with fruits or vegetables for a smoothie, blenders are the very best tools for the job.

Types of blenders

By far, the most popular of all blenders is the traditional, upright blender. Limited improvements have been made to that basic model, but the biggest is the invention of the immersion blender. Cordless and personal-size blenders have made their way onto the market, too, but they've resonated with a relatively small number of consumers.

Traditional, home kitchen blenders

The traditional blender has a tall glass, stainless steel, or plastic container, with a lid sporting a hole in the middle. It sits on a base housing the motor and plug. Blades are attached to the bottom of the container; there may be two or four blades that do the work of cutting food into small particles.

Here are the advantages of traditional blenders for making smoothies:

- The vortex action means that food is liquefied and drinkable.
- You can add softer fruits and vegetables through the opening in the lid toward the end of the blending.
- They're relatively inexpensive, ranging in price from less than $50 to less than $100.

Here are the disadvantages of traditional blenders for making smoothies:

- Food gets caught underneath the small blades.
- If not enough liquid is added to the container, the food may get stuck in the blades and can't be processed.
- Most can't handle ice, grains, coffee beans, spices, and very hard vegetables.

Bottom line: Blenders work better than food processors for making smoothies; they're inexpensive and reliable for simple smoothies and puréed foods but aren't powerful enough to handle ice and hard ingredients.

High-performance blenders

Blenders in this category are called *high performance* for may reasons, most importantly because of the size and power of the motor, which impacts their ability to liquidize fruits and hard root vegetables, chop ice, blend frozen mixtures, mix batter, chop dry ingredients like grains and coffee, and purée nuts for nut butters and raw vegetable dips.

For a long time, the VitaMix brand blender was the only reliable high-performance blender available for home and commercial kitchens. Now, other manufacturers of commercial and home kitchen food prep products are designing and producing blenders that fall into this category. One new feature in some brands is a pre-programmed or timed cycle that lets you walk away from the machine while it blends the ingredients and then automatically shuts off.

I've tested some of the top high-performance blenders available today and compiled Table 3-1 for easy comparison of their features. Keep in mind that many of these brands have several other models with different features that are higher or lower in price, and some may offer certified refurbished machines at considerable savings, so do a bit more research to determine what make and model is best for your price range.

The advantages of high-performance blenders for making smoothies are as follows:

✔ The powerful motor can handle hard fruits and vegetables, as well as grains and nuts.
✔ The size of the container means that you can make more than a few servings at one time.

Bottom line: If you can afford it, this type of blender can get you making not only smoothies, but also soups, frozen drinks, nut butters, and desserts.

Immersion blenders

The immersion or stick blender consists of a slim motor that fits into the handle of a tool that can be gripped with one hand; the mixing and cutting blades are attached to the end of the wand. The name comes from the fact that you can immerse the blade into a bowl of ingredients. Equipped with different speeds, the immersion blender is designed for light-duty blending of light batters, sauces, and dips.

Here are the advantages of immersion blenders for making smoothies:

✔ They're very small and slim — they can fit in a drawer.
✔ They're somewhat portable.

Table 3-1   **Comparing High-Performance Blenders**

Brand	Model	Motor Size	Features	Warranty	Cost Range**
Blendtec (www.blendtec.com) An excellent, high-tech choice Not included but exceptional: Twister Jar for nut butters, thick mixtures, dry grinding	Designer Classic 725	1,560 watts 3.8 HP	100 manual capacitive touch speeds; five pre-programmed, timed cycles; self-clean cycle; 96 oz. jug; metal drive coupling; touch-pad controls guide you through set-up and beyond; best spatula for removing food from jug	8 years	High Other models available ranging low to medium
Breville (www.breville.com) An excellent choice	The Boss	1,500 watts 2 HP	12 manual speeds; five pre-programmed, timed cycles; self-clean cycle; 68 oz. heavy-duty jug for wet and dry ingredients; metal drive coupling; flex spatula; beautiful hardcover recipe book	7 years	Medium
Hamilton Beach (commercial.hamiltonbeach.com) A commercial machine moving into consumer market, a good machine	HBH650 Series Tempest	880 watts 3 HP	Two manual speeds; timer with automatic shutoff; 64 oz. jug; metal drive coupling; unique jug shape forces ingredients into the blades, making ice and hard ingredients liquefy faster	2 years	High

(continued)

Table 3-1 (continued)

Brand	Model	Motor Size	Features	Warranty	Cost Range**
Omni (www.3blenders.com) Excellent value for the cost	OmniBlend V	950 watts 3 HP	Three manual touch speeds; three timed settings with automatic shutoff; 64 oz. jug; metal drive coupling	7 years	Low
VitaMix (www.vitamix.com) Still reliable and excellent value considering the dry grains jug is included	C-Series 5200	1380 watts 2 HP	Variable dial speed; 64 oz jug and 32 oz. dry grains jug; metal drive coupling; excellent recipe book	7 years	Medium Several models available

**Cost ranges according to list prices: Low: $250 to $349; Medium: $350 to $549; High: $550 to $700+

Here are the disadvantages of immersion blenders for making smoothies:

- ✔ They can't crush ice.
- ✔ They can't blend harder fruits and vegetables.

Bottom line: An immersion blender may come in handy if you're making mashed potatoes, sauces, or dips, but when it comes to making smoothies, an immersion blender isn't up for the job.

Features to look for in a blender

Blenders are so ubiquitous that people sometimes forget that there are different features that make each make and model unique. If you plan to make smoothies daily, you'll want to keep the blender on top of the counter, so height, size, and appearance will be a consideration in addition to the features outlined in this section.

Container material and size

Blender containers are made from

- ✔ **Plastic:** The least expensive blender containers are made from plastic. The advantages of plastic are that it's lightweight and chip-proof.
- ✔ **Glass:** Glass is durable and won't discolor or absorb odors from herbs or vegetables the way plastic can.
- ✔ **Stainless steel:** Stainless steel is the most expensive and the most durable. It keeps frozen mixtures cold longer. On the downside, you can't see the mixture inside until you take the lid off.

Containers range in capacity from 8 ounces for the personal or mini blender container to 10 to 64 ounces for the average traditional blender to 80 ounces for a high-performance blender. Only you can determine what size is appropriate for your needs.

Motor size

As with juicers, the power of the motor is important for blending hard and fibrous vegetables. The average kitchen blender boasts between 300 and 600 watts of power, with the high-performance blenders weighing in at an average, whopping 1,300 watts.

Opt for the most powerful motor you can afford when choosing a blender — the higher the wattage, the more versatile your machine will be. A lower-wattage machine won't be able to handle thick, frozen cocktails; sorbets; and granitas.

Drive socket and blades

Look for stainless steel drive socket, blades, and blade drive shaft because plastic wears out quickly. The drive socket should be easy and inexpensive to replace because it may be stripped if something blocks the blades from turning. This protects the motor from overworking.

Pulsing button

If you plan to make iced drinks, sorbets, or granitas, a pulsing button is essential. The ice falls into the blades when paused and is ground up again when the blades begin to spin. Without the pulsing button on your blender, you will have to stop and mix up the ice before starting the motor again.

Variable speeds

Being able to start the blender at a slow speed and gradually increase it to high puts less stress on the motor. The ability to reduce from a high speed to a very low speed allows you to add ingredients at the end of blending that you don't want to be liquidized or puréed into the rest of the mixture.

Ice crusher

This function is similar to the pulsing button. It automatically stops and restarts the blades so that ice can be easily chopped and integrated evenly into a blended mixture.

Cleaning Your Juicer or Blender

Always, always, always clean your juicer or blender immediately after you use it — as soon as the drink has been poured into glasses and before you sit down to enjoy it. The natural sugars in fruits and vegetables can make cleaning the equipment a nightmare if you wait — they're sticky and cause the smaller particles of liquid and other ingredients to adhere (like glue) to the lid, the container, the blades, and any utensil or surface that the mixture has been spilled on or otherwise touched.

Cleaning a juicer

To clean a juicer, follow these steps:

1. **Fill the sink with hot, soapy water.**

   You can do this before you even start juicing, after you've washed and scrubbed the produce.

2. After you've processed the food and poured the juice into a glass, unplug the juicer and disassemble the machine, immersing the parts into the hot, soapy water.

3. Using a brush, clean each part and rinse it under hot water.

4. Wipe down the motor base and the countertop where you've been working with a hot, soapy cloth.

5. Let the parts dry while you enjoy your juice.

6. After the parts are dry, reassemble the juicer so the machine is ready for your next healthy drink.

Cleaning a blender

To clean a blender, follow these steps:

1. After you've processed the food and poured the smoothie into a glass, rinse out the container.

2. Add a few drops of liquid soap to the container, and fill it one-quarter to one-half full of hot water.

3. Place the lid on the container and blend, starting at low and moving to high speed, and then back down to low.

4. Turn off the machine, unplug it, and pour the soapy water over the inside of the lid and into the sink.

5. Rinse the container and the lid with hot water.

6. Wipe down the motor base and the countertop where you've been working with a hot, soapy cloth.

Chapter 4

Stocking Up to Make Juices and Smoothies

*P*lanning saves you money, as well as time, and it keeps you organized so that making juices and smoothies can be a seamless part of your daily routine. Planning what to shop for keeps you focused on the juices and smoothies you'll make and helps you to organize the ingredients you have on hand and those you need to purchase. Planning when and where you'll shop lets you work market days into a routine that suits your work and leisure activities.

In general, you should use fresh fruits and vegetables within two or three days of purchase. That's why you'll want to plan how, when, where, and what to buy — one big grocery outing every week just won't work.

This chapter is all about buying and handling fresh fruits and vegetables, what to look for when shopping, how to treat them so that their nutrients are retained, and making sure that you get the benefit of optimum nutrition when you use them in juices or smoothies.

Your excursion into healthy drinks starts with the recipes and a list of what you need for a few days' refreshment. After you get into the habit of list making and planning a few days' drink recipes, you'll wonder how you ever survived without these valuable habits — and you may find it helpful to transfer those habits to meal planning and shopping, too.

Shopping Like a Pro

A peach is a peach is a peach, right? Not exactly. The quality of the nutrients in the peach you place into your grocery cart depends on many things, including what variety of peach it is, where and in what kind of soil it was grown, at what stage in its maturity it was picked, how far and in what kind of container it had to travel to get to the store, how long it's been sitting on the produce shelf, and whether it was subjected to regular misting with water before you plucked it.

The goal is to choose fresh, local organic produce that's in season where you live. This commitment serves both you and your local food community. Here's how: You get fruits and vegetables that have ripened on the vine or tree (instead of being picked green and ripened with gas) and developed their full complement of vitamins, minerals, and phytonutrients, and you support the growers in your area so that they can keep growing vital crops.

Making a list and checking it twice

Organized people live by their lists. They are "thinking" shoppers who take advantage of produce that is ripe and in season because it's the most economical and at its peak. Here's what a shopping list does for you:

- **It keeps you on track.** Your goal to look and feel better is achievable if you aim for the optimum number of servings of a wide variety of fruits and vegetables every day. Making a list motivates you to make healthy choices, choose a wide variety of fruit and vegetable recipes, and stick to their ingredient lists when shopping.

- **It saves you money.** Planning the recipes and noting the fruits and vegetables and other ingredients you have on hand before you leave for the store means that you won't come home with something you already have or don't need. And it saves you an extra trip back to the store for something you missed.

- **It keeps you from getting into a rut.** Making a list before you shop encourages you to check out new recipes so that you step out of your normal favorites. It widens your perspective and gives you new ingredients from which to choose instead of relying on the same three or four items.

- **It helps you plan where and when you'll shop.** All food spoils, but making a list and shopping for two or three days' worth of ingredients means your fresh produce is always at its peak for juicing and smoothies.

✔ **It saves you time and effort.** Making a list may seem like more work at first, but when you go into the market you won't waste time going up and down the aisles or wandering around the produce section wondering what to buy. Produce shopping every two or three days means that your cart is lighter and you can get in and out, pack the car, and be gone in record time.

Knowing what to look for in produce

You're focused on your health (otherwise, you wouldn't be reading this book). So, it stands to reason that you want to start with the finest produce so that you get the highest-quality vitamins, minerals, and phytonutrients. Don't compromise. Get the freshest fruits and vegetables you can find. Here's how:

✔ **Shop for organic produce.** There's a reason why certified organic food production is growing all over the world. Actually, there are several reasons, and they have to do with the health of the planet and the health of people. There is concrete scientific evidence that organic farming results in

- Healthier soil

- Less soil erosion

- Cleaner waterways

- Reduction in human and wildlife exposure to persistent toxic chemicals

- Less energy usage than conventional farming — 30 percent to 50 percent less

- A healthy population of birds and insects in and around the farm

Fresh organic produce yields more nutrients because you don't need to peel it. Many of the vitamins, minerals, and phytonutrients in fruits and vegetables are concentrated in and just below the peel or skin, but that's exactly where chemical pesticides and herbicides are lurking.

Although North American countries have banned the use of certain toxic pesticides (such as DDT), those chemicals are still being produced and exported to food-producing countries and coming back to us in fruits and vegetables. If non-organic is your only option, at least try to avoid the following "dirty dozen" — these fruits and vegetables have the highest concentrations of pesticides: apples, bell peppers, blueberries (domestic, not wild), celery, grapes (especially if imported), kale/collard greens, lettuce, nectarines, peaches, potatoes, spinach, and strawberries.

If you have no choice but to purchase non-organic produce, always peel it if you want to reduce pesticide exposure.

✔ **Shop for produce that's in season.** The term *in season* means that, where you live, the crops grown locally are being harvested *right now*. Because of this, plenty of those fruits or vegetables are available, at the lowest prices, and they're fresher than imports. If they're grown locally, fruits and vegetables will have ripened naturally, on the vine or on the tree, and their nutrients will be higher than produce that's picked before it's ripe and transported in refrigerated crates.

To find out what's in season when, check out Fruits & Veggies—More Matters (`www.fruitsandveggiesmorematters.org/what-fruits-and-vegetables-are-in-season`).

✔ **Plan to use what's in season.** This means using, among other things, tomatoes and peaches in the summer, apples and cranberries in the fall, winter pears and cabbage in the winter, and leafy greens and asparagus in the spring. Unless you live in tropical areas, winter strawberries and tomatoes aren't the best choice for flavor, nutrients, or price. If you want to use strawberries in winter, plan to pick your own at a local farm in the summer and freeze them for winter smoothies.

✔ **Get it from the person who grows it.** Many farmers sell right on the premises in farm gate sales, because it saves them time, energy, and transportation costs. If you buy directly from the farmer, the fruits and vegetables will be fresh picked and at their peak. They will have ripened the way nature intended, and they'll be bursting with vitamins, minerals, and phytonutrients because they matured properly.

If you can't make a trip to a nearby farm (or if farms are too far from where you live), you may be able to buy from the farmers at your local farmers' market.

Don't be fooled by "fake" farmers at the farmers' market. Some markets are very strict about only inviting the person who raises the fruits or vegetables; others allow middlemen (people who just buy and sell food, as opposed to growing it). You can't miss the fake farmers — their produce comes in boxes labeled "produce of" followed by the name of some faraway place.

✔ **Grow your own.** Growing your own vegetables isn't all that hard, and it can be done in very small spaces. You can grow vegetables in containers on a balcony or on very small patches of land. For more information, check out *Container Gardening For Dummies,* 2nd Edition, by Bill Marken, Suzanne DeJohn, and the editors of the National Gardening Association (John Wiley & Sons, Inc.).

✔ **Know how to tell if it's fresh.** A light touch on peaches, plums, avocadoes, and melons can easily help gauge their ripeness. Most fruit smells sweet and fragrant when ripe, so go ahead and give it a sniff and a gentle caress. Be aware of the difference between fresh, in-season specials and the discount bin, which is food that is past its prime. Produce from the discount bin may be tempting due to its price, but it'll be past its peak, and many of the nutrients will have been lost.

Weighing your options: Fresh, dried, frozen, or canned

When you're buying fruits and vegetables, you have four basic options: fresh dried, frozen, and canned. Which has the best quality? And are the others close or far behind?

✔ **Fresh:** Hands down, fresh is always best when you can buy it directly from the farm or when it's locally grown and in season. Fresh fruit has less nutrients if it's immature (under-ripe or picked before it ripens) or over-ripe (past its peak). The quality of fresh fruit declines the farther it has to travel to get to your table.

The United States Department of Agriculture (USDA) has prepared two excellent online resources, "How to Buy Fresh Fruits" (`www.ams.usda.gov/AMSv1.0/getfile?dDocName=STELDEV3103620`) and "How to Buy Fresh Vegetables" (`www.ams.usda.gov/AMSv1.0/getfile?dDocName=STELDEV3103623`), which give information on quality, nutrition, labeling, grades, and how to select specific fruits and vegetables.

✔ **Dried:** Dried fruits and vegetables have only had the water removed — all the nutrients should be intact unless heat was used in the drying process and an excess amount of sugar was added (which degrades the nutrients). In the winter, you may want to use dried fruits in smoothies.

If heat was used in the drying process, the label will show sugar as an added ingredient, and it may list the drying process used.

If fruit is dried chemically by adding preservatives such as sulfur dioxide, it isn't a healthy choice, so look for *unsulfured* dried fruit. It will be brown and not as visually appealing, but it's much healthier.

✔ **Frozen:** Local, in-season fresh fruits and vegetables are best, but frozen is next to best — and in some cases, frozen is actually the better choice. This is because fruits and vegetables that are commercially frozen tend to be processed close to where they grew and at their peak ripeness, a time when they're most packed with nutrients. Of course, buying local fresh fruits and vegetables and freezing your own is the very best way to ensure that you'll have those strawberries for winter smoothies.

✔ **Canned:** A canned fruit or vegetable is better than none at all. So, if your teenager wants a peach smoothie after school, go right ahead and stock the pantry with canned peaches if you haven't frozen your own.

Canned tomatoes, pumpkin and legumes (beans and peas) retain most of their life-giving nutrients, so keeping cans of these organic vegetables in your pantry is a good idea.

So, if fresh is best, why even mention canned or frozen? Local fresh produce is available only once, perhaps twice, a year, depending on where you live. Plus, if you grow your own, you know that you can't keep up with the amount your garden is producing, even if you're juicing every day. Add to that the fact that you really should be including berries and a wide range of summer-only fruits and vegetables in your diet and, well, you see the dilemma. It makes sense to use some canned and frozen produce to augment the fresh winter local produce available where you live.

Treating Fruits and Vegetables like Gold

What you do with fruits and vegetables when they're in your hands is as important as all the steps that took place long before you saw them. After you choose that fruit or vegetable, it's up to you to handle it as if it were gold. After you place fresh produce into your grocery cart, it's up to you to wash, store, and use it with care so that you benefit from the optimum nutrients.

Transporting fruits and veggies

You've gone to the farm or the farmers' market or bought local produce at the supermarket. To get fresh produce home without compromising its fresh state or the nutrients it contains, do the following:

✔ **Keep insulated bags or a cooler in the car and put the fruits and vegetables in them.** Wilting and loss of some nutrients start immediately after picking and during the trip home in a hot trunk or back seat.

✔ **Head straight home after buying the most perishable foods.** Some foods, like apples, carrots, and pears, will last longer, but don't plan on running any more errands after you pick up more delicate greens, berries, peaches, and stone fruits.

✔ **Make produce runs first thing in the morning or in the cooler evenings during the summer months whenever possible.**

Cleaning your fruits and veggies

It's a myth that organic foods don't need to be washed. Think about that turnip pushing its pointy head up through the soil. If that turnip is lucky enough to be growing in organic soil, that soil is bursting with microbes, bacteria, and other helpful soil organisms. And that turnip will pass through several hands (perhaps even be sneezed on) before it finds its way to your grocery cart.

It's a fact: Bacteria such as listeria, salmonella, and *E. coli* may be clinging to your fruits and vegetables. Washing is the first line of defense in protecting the produce — and you — so here are some tips:

✔ **Wash firm fruits and root vegetables, celery, apples, grapes, and stone fruits when you get home from the market.** That way, you can set these healthy foods out as snacks and know that they won't have nasty chemicals or bacteria to cause food-borne illness.

✔ **Don't wash delicate foods such as berries and mushrooms until just before you're ready to use them.** This keeps them dry and helps prevent mold from working its destruction.

✔ **Wash all pre-packaged fruits and vegetables, even if the label claims they have been pre-washed.** One of the easiest and most effective ways to clean most vegetables, as well as tree and stone fruit, is to immerse them in a sink full of cool water with ¼ cup white vinegar added. Use a vegetable brush to gently scrub them all over. Rinse and pat dry before storing. Wash delicate fruit such as raspberries, strawberries, and blueberries by placing them in a colander or sieve and swishing them through the vinegar water. Rinse and pat dry before using.

Never use soaps, detergents, bleaches or other toxic cleaning chemicals on your precious produce. These chemicals will leave a toxic residue of their own.

Figure 4-1 shows how to wash your fruits and veggies so they're clean and ready for your juices and smoothies.

Figure 4-1:
Washing your fruits and vegetables.

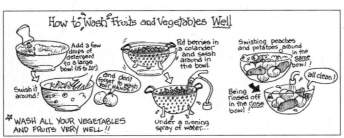

Illustration by Elizabeth Kurtzman

Storing your fruits and veggies

Storing fruits and vegetables properly will save you money because they'll stay fresh until you use them. Use the information in Table 4-1 to safely store that precious commodity.

Table 4-1		Storing Fruits and Vegetables		
Fruit or Vegetable	**Refrigerate in the Crisper Drawer up to Seven Days**	**Store on the Countertop out of Direct Sunlight up to Seven Days**	**Store in a Cool, Dry, Dark Place for Three to Six Months**	**Ripen on the Counter and Refrigerate When Ripe up to Seven days**
Apples*		X	X	
Apricots (fresh)*	X			
Artichokes	X			
Asparagus	X			
Avocadoes*				X
Bananas*		X		
Beets	X			
Berries (unwashed)	X			
Broccoli	X			
Brussels sprouts	X			
Cabbage	X			
Carrots	X			
Cauliflower	X			
Celery	X			
Cherries	X			
Corn (in the husk, unwashed)	X			
Cucumbers		X		
Eggplant		X		

Fruit or Vegetable	Refrigerate in the Crisper Drawer up to Seven Days	Store on the Countertop out of Direct Sunlight up to Seven Days	Store in a Cool, Dry, Dark Place for Three to Six Months	Ripen on the Counter and Refrigerate When Ripe up to Seven days
Figs (fresh)*	X			
Garlic (in a net bag; hung in a well-ventilated, cool place)			X	
Grapes	X			
Green beans	X			
Green onions	X			
Greens (unwashed)	X			
Herbs (washed, in a clean cloth)	X			
Kiwifruit				X
Melons*	X			
Mushrooms (unwashed, in a paper bag)	X			
Nectarines*				X
Onions (in a net bag; hung in a well-ventilated, cool place)			X	
Peaches*				X
Pears*				X
Plums				X

(continued)

Table 4-1 *(continued)*

Fruit or Vegetable	Refrigerate in the Crisper Drawer up to Seven Days	Store on the Countertop out of Direct Sunlight up to Seven Days	Store in a Cool, Dry, Dark Place for Three to Six Months	Ripen on the Counter and Refrigerate When Ripe up to Seven days
Potatoes			X	
Pumpkins			X	
Radishes	X			
Summer squash	X			
Sweet potatoes			X	
Tomatoes*		X		
Winter squash			X	

*Give off excessive amounts of ethylene gas, which speeds up the ripening process of the fruits and vegetables around them. Store away from other produce, never in the same bowl, bag, or drawer.

Freezing them for the future

Freezing fruits and vegetables when they're at their peak is one of the easiest ways to preserve them for use later. If you grow or pick your own or purchase fruits and vegetables when in season and in quantity, you can save a considerable amount of money in the winter, when the same produce is being transported from warm climates.

Using frozen fruit in smoothies makes the drink thick and icy cold. You can partially thaw fruit and vegetables before juicing them and the result will be thick and creamy. Here is the best way to freeze the most common fruits and vegetables.

Berries

To freeze berries, such as blackberries, blueberries, currants, raspberries, and strawberries, follow these steps:

1. **Wash, hull, or de-stem the berries and dry.**

2. **Place them in a single layer on baking sheets, and freeze them for one to two hours.**

3. Measure 1- or 2-cup amounts into freezer bags, label the bags, and freeze.

   Store for up to three to six months.

Stone fruit

To freeze stone fruit, such as apricots, cherries, mangoes, nectarines, peaches, and plums, follow these steps:

1. **Wash, halve, remove the stone or pit, and cut into smaller pieces.**
2. **For each cup of light-fleshed fruit (like peaches or mangoes), toss the pieces in 2 tablespoons of lemon juice.**
3. **Place in a single layer on baking sheets, and freeze for one to two hours.**
4. **Measure 1- or 2-cup amounts into freezer bags, label the bags, and freeze.**

   Store for up to three to six months.

Tree fruit

To freeze tree fruit, such as apples, bananas, citrus fruit, guavas, kiwifruit, medlar, or pears, follow these steps:

1. **Wash, peel (if citrus or bananas), quarter, remove the core, and cut the quarters in half.**
2. **For each cup of fruit, toss the pieces in 2 tablespoons of lemon juice.**
3. **Place in a single layer on baking sheets, and freeze for one to two hours.**
4. **Measure 1- or 2-cup amounts into freezer bags, label the bags, and freeze.**

   Store for up to six to nine months.

Vegetables (hard)

To freeze hard vegetables, such as beets, carrots, celery, onions, parsnips, peppers, rutabaga, turnips, or winter squash, follow these steps:

1. **Wash, pat dry, and cut into 1- or 2-inch pieces.**
2. **Measure 2- or 4-cup amounts into freezer bags, label the bags, and freeze.**

   Store for up to 9 to 12 months.

Vegetables (medium)

To freeze medium vegetables, such as asparagus, beans, broccoli, Brussels sprouts, cauliflower, or peas, follow these steps:

1. **Wash, trim, sort, or cut into uniform sizes.**

2. **Leave whole or cut into 2-inch lengths.**

3. **Blanch in boiling water for 3 minutes, and then plunge into cold water for 3 minutes.**

4. **Pat dry and place in freezer bags, label the bags, and freeze.**

   Store for up to six to nine months.

Greens

To freeze greens, such as beet greens, collards, kale, mustard greens, spinach, Swiss chard, or turnip greens, follow these steps:

1. **Remove tough stems and imperfect leaves.**

2. **Blanch in boiling water for 2 minutes, and then plunge into cold water for 2 minutes.**

3. **Pat dry, coarsely chop, and place in freezer bags; label the bags; and freeze.**

   Store for up to four to six months.

Part II

Liquid Gold: The Health Benefits of Juicing and Smoothies

Four benefits from going with a liquid lifestyle

- ✔ Eliminate high-fat and high-calorie foods that only add calories with no nutrients.
- ✔ Reset your taste sensors to eliminate your craving for salty or sugar-filled junk food.
- ✔ Add valuable fiber to help your body eliminate toxins and keep you regular.
- ✔ Flood your cells with high-quality nutrients that repair cells and protect against diseases.

Check out www.dummies.com/extras/juicingsmoothies for how to live the juicing and smoothie lifestyle.

In this part . . .

- ✔ Examine all the incredible health benefits that juices and smoothies offer so that you can incorporate drinking more of them on a daily basis.

- ✔ Look closer at the kinds of rewards your body will reap — on the inside as well as the outside by drinking juices and smoothies.

- ✔ Optimize health habits by tailoring juices and smoothies throughout your life cycle, starting with your children and all the way to your senior years.

- ✔ Discover how to prevent modern diseases, such as diabetes, heart disease, and cancers by increasing fruits and vegetables in your daily diet with juices and smoothies.

- ✔ Detox and cleanse your body with juices to eliminate toxins, impurities, and free radicals so that you can eliminate feeling sluggish.

Chapter 5

Science and Nutrition in a Glass

*A*s science and technology bring more detailed information about the foods that people eat, the crucial role of nutrition in the maintenance of good health becomes increasingly clear. Along with the growing trove of information about nutrition is the knowledge about what kinds of foods provide the very best nutrients. So, the key to good health is twofold:

✔ Eat as wide a range as possible of the nutrients your body needs in order to function at its best.

✔ Find organic, whole foods that provide the best-quality nutrients.

Juices and smoothies are an important part of a whole-foods diet because they allow you to get an above-average quota of fresh fruits and vegetables and, thus, fiber, macronutrients (protein, fat, and carbohydrates), and micronutrients (vitamins, minerals, and so on) every day.

This chapter fills you in on the nature and role of all the essential nutrients that you can get from food. With this information, you can design your juicing and smoothies program so that you draw from a wide rainbow of fruits and vegetables.

For much more information on nutrition, be sure to check out the latest edition of *Nutrition For Dummies* by Carol Ann Rinzler (John Wiley & Sons, Inc.).

Focusing on Vitamins

Vitamins are organic food substances found only in plants and animals.
They're essential for growth, energy, and tissue maintenance, as well as for
a whole list of specific functions your body performs. With the exception of
vitamin D, your body cannot manufacture vitamins, so you have to get them
from the foods you eat. Table 5-1 outlines the vitamins, what they do for
your body, what happens if you don't get enough of them, and which juice or
smoothie ingredients are good sources of those vitamins.

Table 5-1		Vitamins	
Vitamin	**What It Does for Your Body**	**What Happens if You Don't Get Enough**	**Best Smoothie/ Juice Ingredients**
Vitamin A	Provides healthy skin, hair, and body tissue; boosts immunity; aids vision; promotes bone and tooth growth	Colds, infections, dry skin, rashes, acne, night blindness, poor bone growth, weak tooth enamel	Apricots, cantaloupe, carrots, guava, kale, mango, papaya, peaches, spinach, squash, sweet potato
Vitamin B1	Helps cells convert carbohydrates into energy; assists digestion; improves brain and heart function, muscles, and nervous system	Weakness and fatigue, lack of concentration, stomach problems, poor digestion	Asparagus, flaxseed, legumes, mangos, milk, oatmeal, peppers, pineapple, sesame seeds, soy milk, sunflower seeds, tomatoes, yogurt
Vitamin B2	Releases energy from protein, fats, and carbohydrates; provides healthy skin, hair, and nails; assists cell growth and reproduction; helps red blood cell production	Lack of energy; dull hair and skin; eczema; dry, cracked lips	Almonds, bean sprouts, broccoli, Brussels sprouts, dates, legumes, mango, milk, soybeans, soy milk, spinach, wheat germ, yogurt

Vitamin	What It Does for Your Body	What Happens if You Don't Get Enough	Best Smoothie/ Juice Ingredients
Vitamin B3	Promotes normal brain function, facilitates digestion, produces energy, provides healthy skin	Headaches, anxiety, depression, insomnia, stomach problems, skin problems	Avocados, guava, legumes, mangos, nectarines, parsnip, peaches, peas, pumpkin, spirulina, squash
Vitamin B5	Metabolizes food, forms hormones and good cholesterol, provides healthy skin and hair, maintains brain and nerves	Low energy, muscle cramps, nausea	Avocados, broccoli, collard greens, corn, oatmeal, raspberries, spirulina, squash, sweet potatoes, yogurt
Vitamin B6	Assists in protein digestion, balances sex hormones, boosts immunity and red blood cell production, helps nerve function	Poor digestion, nausea, dizziness, confusion, depression, irritability, convulsions	Avocados, bananas, broccoli, corn, green pepper, hazelnuts, legumes, pumpkin seeds, spinach, squash, sunflower seeds, walnuts
Vitamin B9	Helps production of red blood cells, helps brain and nervous system activity, plays a crucial part in spinal fluid, essential for pregnant women and fetuses	Anemia, anxiety, depression, exhaustion, skin problems	Broccoli, cashews, collard greens, legumes, lentils, mangos, papayas, peanuts, peas, sesame seeds, spinach, turnip greens, walnuts, wheat germ, yogurt
Vitamin B12	Assists in formation of blood cells, promotes metabolism, helps insulate the nerves	Tiredness, irritability, anemia	Cheddar cheese, cottage cheese, milk, yogurt

(continued)

Table 5-1 *(Continued)*

Vitamin	What It Does for Your Body	What Happens if You Don't Get Enough	Best Smoothie/ Juice Ingredients
Vitamin C	Protects body tissue from oxidation damage, fights infection, provides strong bones and teeth, aids in the absorption of iron	Colds, flu, infections, slow healing of cuts and bruises, skin problems, cancer, cardiovascular disease	Broccoli, Brussels sprouts, cantaloupe, citrus fruit, kale, kiwi, mangos, papayas, peppers, pineapples, squash, strawberries, Swiss chard
Vitamin D	Promotes absorption of calcium and magnesium for strong teeth and bones	Stiff, painful joints; tooth decay; leg pain; low immunity; low energy; fatigue	Milk*
Vitamin E	Is a powerful antioxidant, assists in the formation of red blood cells, prevents scarring, soothes and heals stressed skin tissue	Exhaustion, atherosclerosis, slow healing of wounds	Almonds, asparagus, bell peppers, mangos, nuts, papayas, pomegranates, spinach, squash, sunflower seeds, Swiss chard, turnip greens, wheat germ
Vitamin K	Plays a role in blood clotting, regulates blood calcium levels, aids bone health	Easy bleeding, weak bones	Alfalfa sprouts, blackberries, blueberries, broccoli, Brussels sprouts, cabbage, cranberries, kale, kiwis, parsley, plums, spinach, Swiss chard

*The body manufactures vitamin D after sun exposure.

Identifying Minerals

Minerals are tiny organic elements that you need to keep your body working properly in order to be healthy. Minerals originate *only* in the soil; plants and animals (including humans) do not create minerals. Instead, plants must absorb minerals from the soil, and animals must get them from plants or other animals.

Smoothies and juices that are made from fresh, local, organic, *raw* fruits and vegetables contain the most live enzymes, vitamins, minerals, and *phytonutrients* (nutrients found in plants — they're not essential the way vitamins and minerals are, but they're still good for you). Minerals vary with geographic location (where your food is grown). One of the advantages of organic soil is that it tends to be richer in minerals than non-organic soil. Minerals (and other phytonutrients) are lost when food is transported over long distances or when it isn't stored properly. Because cooking destroys some minerals and vitamins, it's best to eat or drink raw fruits and vegetables.

Like everything in life, the various functions and workings of minerals are complicated. Some must be present for breaking down, digesting, absorbing, and releasing energy from food — these are the minerals that are important for energy. Some help to strengthen bones, muscles, nails, and teeth. Some regulate water and cholesterol in the body. Some minerals work at their peak when other minerals or vitamins are present, while other minerals are hindered by the presence of some vitamins.

If you eat a wide range of fruits and vegetables and combine them with other whole foods (such as legumes, nuts, seeds, herbs, and low-fat milk products), you can get all the vitamins and minerals you need for optimum health.

Table 5-2 outlines the minerals, what they do for your body, what happens if you don't get enough of them, and which juice or smoothie ingredients are good sources of those minerals.

Table 5-2		Minerals	
Mineral	*What It Does for Your Body*	*What Happens if You Don't Get Enough*	*Best Smoothie/ Juice Ingredients*
Calcium	Eases insomnia, helps nutrients get into the blood, builds healthy muscles, aids in blood clotting, assists nerves in transmitting information	Weak bones, osteoporosis, muscle spasms, cramps, insomnia, high blood pressure	Almonds, blackberries, broccoli, dates, kale, kelp, milk, molasses, papayas, sesame seeds, spinach, tofu, yogurt

(continued)

Table 5-2 *(Continued)*

Mineral	What It Does for Your Body	What Happens if You Don't Get Enough	Best Smoothie/ Juice Ingredients
Chromium	Balances blood sugar and heart activity	Irritability, drowsiness	Apples, oats, onions, tomatoes, wheat germ
Iron	Boosts energy, assists in carrying oxygen in the blood	Anemia, fatigue	Cherries, figs, kale, legumes, lentils, lima beans, sesame seeds, soybeans, spinach, squash, strawberries, Swiss chard, tofu
Magnesium	Promotes strong teeth and bones, promotes new cell growth, activates B vitamins, assists in absorption of calcium and vitamin C, boosts energy	Fatigue, nervousness, insomnia, heart problems, high blood pressure, muscle weakness, cramps	Bananas, garlic, nuts, pumpkin seeds, raisins, sesame seeds, soybeans, spinach, squash, sunflower seeds, Swiss chard, wheat germ
Manganese	Promotes healthy bones, protects cells from free radical damage, promotes optimum function of thyroid, aids insulin production, maintains health of tissues and nerves	Dizziness, fits, painful joints	Bananas, beets, legumes, nuts, oats, pineapples, pumpkin seeds, raspberries, spinach, strawberries, watercress
Phosphorous	Promotes healthy bones, teeth, and nerve cells; boosts energy	Bone fractures, muscle weakness	Almost all fruits and vegetables
Potassium	Helps sodium regulate water balance, ensures healthy heart function, assists nutrient absorption, helps muscles contract and relax, boosts nerve reflexes	Irregular heartbeat, muscle weakness, nausea, low blood pressure, cellulite, irritability	Almonds, bananas, celery, legumes, lentils, lima beans, milk, papayas, potatoes, pumpkin, pumpkin seeds, radishes, spinach, Swiss chard

Mineral	What It Does for Your Body	What Happens if You Don't Get Enough	Best Smoothie/ Juice Ingredients
Sodium	Works with potassium to regulate water balance, regulates nerve and heart activity	Dizziness, low blood pressure, nausea, low energy	Beets, celery, cheese, fennel, kale, legumes, milk, watercress, yogurt
Selenium	Protects cells from free radical damage, works with vitamin E	Rare in humans	Asparagus, bananas, cashews, coconuts, guavas, legumes, mangos, parsnip, pomegranates
Zinc	Heals tissue, regulates hormones, aids in stress management, contributes to a healthy nervous system	Infections, acne, greasy skin, depression, loss of appetite	Cheddar cheese, legumes, nuts, oats, pumpkin seeds, sesame seeds, spirulina, Swiss chard

Boosting calcium

Most people think of milk as the best source of calcium — and milk *is* a good source: One 8-ounce glass of 2 percent milk supplies 120 mg of it. But for people who are lactose intolerant, who don't drink a lot of milk, or who can't digest cheese, there are excellent calcium-rich ingredients to add to smoothies or to stir into juices. Here are some foods to use in smoothies or juice to boost your calcium intake:

✔ **Almonds:** 1 ounce of almonds (approximately 23 nuts) has 75 mg calcium. Add it to smoothies.

✔ **Blackstrap molasses:** 1 tablespoon has 137 mg of calcium. Stir it into the juice or add it to ingredients in smoothies.

✔ **Collard greens:** 1 cup of collard greens has 266 mg of calcium. Juice it raw or add it raw or lightly steamed to smoothies.

✔ **Kale:** 1 cup of boiled kale has 94 mg of calcium. Juice it raw or add it raw or lightly steamed to smoothies.

✔ **Papaya:** 1 medium papaya has 73 mg of calcium. It's great juiced or in smoothies.

✔ **Sesame seeds:** ¼ cup has 351 mg of calcium. You can add sesame seeds to smoothies.

✔ **Spinach:** 1 cup of boiled spinach has 245 mg of calcium. Juice it raw or add it raw or lightly steamed to smoothies.

✔ **Seaweed:** 1 cup of raw kelp has 136 mg of calcium (more than a glass of milk). It's best rehydrated and used in smoothies.

✔ **Tahini:** 2 tablespoons raw tahini (sesame seed butter) has 126 mg of calcium. Add it to smoothie ingredients.

Examining Enzymes

Enzymes are chemicals produced by your glands and released into the bloodstream. Think of them as your body's couriers, surfing the blood to get to their destinations with top priority or life-changing messages.

Enzymes are released by various endocrine glands — the pituitary, hypothalamus, and thyroid glands, for example — and travel through your bloodstream to reach their target organs or tissues where they trigger some specific action by that part of the body. In this way, enzymes facilitate proper functioning of your body in areas of growth, development, and reproduction.

In addition to being produced by your own glands, enzymes are produced in plants and animals. The enzymes in *live* or raw plants are best used in smoothies or juices (or eaten raw) so that they can do their job as messengers and save your body from the work of producing them.

Recognizing what enzymes do

Enzymes are simply messengers. They don't actually do anything except deliver information to specific parts of your body in order for them to do something. So, the cells or organs react to the chemical stimulation carried by the enzymes. Here's what enzymes tell your body to do:

- ✔ Make you grow and stop growing.
- ✔ Make you feel happy or sad.
- ✔ Speed up or slow down your body's metabolism.
- ✔ Start puberty and menopause.
- ✔ Regulate your fighting, mating, and fleeing instincts.

Enzymes are essential to normal growth, development, and reproduction.

Discovering the raw truth

Because enzymes are the keys that trigger the active work of the body, they're critical to good health. Although the body does produce enzymes, outside the body, enzymes are found in all living things,

---

Phytonutrients: Nature's miracle workers

Phytonutrients are natural substances that are found in plants. These tiny, life-giving nutrients can prevent or even cure disease.

"Sign me up!" you say. Well, if you eat and drink a wide range of colorful fruits and vegetables along with whole foods, you'll be getting all the essential nutrients, including phytonutrients, that you need to be well.

If you want more information on phytonutrients, check out *Meals That Heal: A Neutraceutical Approach to Diet and Health,* by Lisa Turner (Healing Arts Press).

---

including food in its raw, uncooked form. Because you can't eat many animal products raw, the very best outside source of enzymes is in fresh, local, organic, raw fruit and vegetables, herbs, grains, legumes, and nuts and seeds.

You should eat a wide range of fruits and vegetables because each food contains the specific enzymes that help break down the elements found within it. For example, the enzyme *amylase* breaks down carbohydrates; amylase is present in bananas, which are high in carbohydrates.

Many people are proponents of a partial or total raw food diet, and many books and other resources are available on the topic. A good general rule is to try to incorporate at least 25 percent raw foods into your overall diet, and the easiest way to do that is by making juices and smoothies every day.

When foods are eaten raw, the food enzymes within those foods do much of the work of digesting them, saving the body from producing enzymes to do the work.

Looking at Protein

Protein has been called the building blocks of the body. It's what your cells, tissues, and very essence are made from. Proteins have a number of functions in your body, including the following:

- Building and repairing body cells, including muscles, teeth, hair, nails, and bones
- Providing a source of energy
- Keeping your immune system functioning properly
- Controlling many of the important processes in the body related to metabolism

Protein is made up of *essential* and *nonessential amino acids.* The body is able to make its own nonessential amino acids, but essential amino acids must be obtained from food. Foods that contain all the essential amino acids are called *complete proteins.* If one or more essential amino acids are missing in a food, that food is called an *incomplete protein.*

Meat and dairy products are complete proteins, but because of saturated fat, these foods may not be the healthiest. So, nutritionists are exploring plant sources of protein. Most plant sources of protein are incomplete, but when their essential amino acids are *combined,* they provide complete protein.

Soybeans are an excellent plant source of complete protein. Quinoa, hemp seeds, and chia seeds are good sources as well.

Table 5-3 lists the essential amino acids and some plant foods for juicing or smoothies that can supply these important nutrients.

Table 5-3	Essential Amino Acids	
Amino Acid	*What It Does*	*Plant Sources for It*
Leucine	Keeps you alert and awake, boosts energy, and stimulates muscle protein synthesis	Seaweed, soybeans, spirulina
Lysine	Slows aging, aids in body growth and blood circulation, protects the immune system, helps the body absorb calcium	Apricots, avocado, figs, guava, kale, lentils, lettuce, pears, persimmon, plums, pumpkin, spinach, sweet potatoes, turnip greens, watermelon
Methionine	Helps cleanse and regenerate kidney and liver cells, stimulates hair growth	Avocado, bean sprouts, broccoli, cauliflower, legumes, mushroom, nuts, oranges, spinach, tofu
Phenylalanine	Helps the thyroid gland produce the hormone thyroxin	Broccoli, spinach, Swiss chard, turnip greens
Threonine	Stimulates digestion and nutrient assimilation	Seaweed, spirulina, watercress
Tryptophan	Helps to promote red blood cells, healthy skin, and hair; works with B vitamins to calm nerves	Seaweed, sesame seeds, soybeans, spinach, spirulina, watercress
Valine	Activates the brain, aids muscle coordination, calms nerves	Seaweed, spirulina, turnip greens

Here are some great protein boosters that you can use in juices and smoothies:

- **Nuts and seeds:** Nuts and seeds are good sources of protein — for example, ¼ cup of almonds contains about 8 grams. Add up to ¼ cup chopped nuts to smoothies.

- **Oats:** One cup of cooked oatmeal has 6 grams of protein. Add ¼ cup per smoothie serving.

- **Soybeans and other legumes:** Soybeans are complete protein providers, and other legumes (like chickpeas and beans) deliver essential amino acids without fat or cholesterol. Add up to ¼ cup to each smoothie serving.

- **Whey powder:** Whey powder is a high-quality complete protein that delivers essential amino acids without fat or cholesterol. Add 1 tablespoon to each smoothie serving or stir into juice.

- **Yogurt, soft cheeses, and tofu:** All contain complete proteins. Add up to ½ cup to smoothies per serving.

Addressing Fluids

Your body is at least 65 percent water, so staying hydrated is important. Water is present in all cells, but it's a major component of your blood. And because the blood feeds your cells and carries away toxins and waste from metabolism, healthy blood means healthy tissues and cells.

Fresh organic vegetable and fruit juices provide vital pure water to your body, and their nutrients help to cleanse the blood and transfer live plant energy to all parts of your body. Pure juices do this without your liver or kidneys having to work to sift out toxins. Most other beverages — including tea, coffee, sodas, alcoholic drinks, and treated water — contain one or more of the following: sugar, additives, preservatives, chlorine, fluoride, and caffeine. These must be eliminated before the body can use the water in them.

Quenching thirst and replenishing minerals lost through sweating is an important function of fresh, pure juices. For an excellent after-exercise drink, juice the following ingredients:

2 slices watermelon with rind, cut to fit the feed tube

2 stalks celery

½ English cucumber

You can mix the juice with an equal amount of pure water or take it straight. Whisk in 1 teaspoon of turmeric — turmeric is an excellent post-exercise herb because it's anti-inflammatory and reduces post-exercise pain.

The truth about supplements

The dietary supplement industry is a powerful force. It spends millions of dollars on communicating the message that poor nutrition can be fixed by popping pills.

By definition of the Health and Education Act, dietary supplements are

✔ Intended to supplement the diet

✔ Contain one or more ingredients (like vitamins, herbs, amino acids, or their constituents)

✔ Meant to be taken orally

✔ Labeled as dietary supplements

The Food and Drug Administration regulates the manufacturing of supplements and ensures that they are produced in a quality manner, free of contaminants or impurities, and accurately labeled.

The first thing to remember about supplements is that they're meant to *enhance* your diet if there are shortfalls or deficiencies. They aren't intended to, nor can they ever replace nutritious foods. In addition, it's important to know that isolated, chemical replicas of vitamins or minerals or phytonutrients can't come close to offering the complex and interactive array of nutrients in whole foods. Although food scientists have identified many key components of food, there are still unidentified nutrients in foods, and all nutrients work together to provide a total healthy and balanced diet.

The American Dietetic Association recognizes that a small number of people may require supplements because the specific nutrients they need are hard to get in adequate amounts in their diets. These groups of people are

✔ Pregnant women and nursing mothers

✔ Strict vegans or vegetarians

✔ People with food allergies or intolerances

✔ Seniors

Bottom line: Unless you fall into a group at risk, take pure vegetable and fruit juices in place of a multivitamin pill; make a lunch or dinner smoothie instead of a meal replacement liquid product; design your own sports juices that replace lost fluids and minerals and that include foods high in sodium and whisk in 1 teaspoon of powdered turmeric to reduce post-exercise pain; eat a whole-food diet; avoid fast food, refined foods, and empty calorie snacks.

Replenishing electrolytes requires sodium, and you can do this by adding one of the following ingredients to smoothies:

2 tablespoons salted almonds or other nuts/seeds

Pinch of sea salt

¼ cup cottage cheese

Don't wait for thirst to tell you that you need to drink water. By that point, your body is dangerously low in fluids.

Drink the Rainbow: How to Make Sure You Get the Nutrients that You Need

The Greek physician Hippocrates (460 B.C.–c. 370 B.C.) said, "Let your food be your medicine." But that was centuries ago. How can you let your food be your medicine today? The U.S. Surgeon General, Canada's Food Guide, the United Kingdom Food Standards Agency, the Australian Government's Department of Health and Aging, and the National Cancer Institute all agree:

> Eating more fruits and vegetables will reduce the risk of cancer and other modern diseases.

Science shows that fruits and vegetables contain all the vitamins, minerals, enzymes, and other phytonutrients that help prevent cancer, heart disease, arthritis, diabetes, osteoporosis, and stroke. Science has now proven what Hippocrates claimed: What you eat becomes your body and what you drink becomes your blood; your food is your medicine.

Finding it hard to cut out the bad foods you've come to eat without thinking? Try squeezing them out. Snack on fresh fruits and vegetables (or drinks made from them) and nuts and seeds. Fill at least half of your mealtime plate with more fruits, vegetables, and legumes, and let whole grains, organic meats, nuts, seeds, and milk products fill the other half. You shouldn't have room for anything else.

The message is clear: For a healthy body, eat a whole-food diet that consists of fresh organic fruits, vegetables, lentils, legumes, herbs, whole grains, nuts, seeds, and small amounts of meat and low-fat dairy products. Using fresh, organic vegetables and fruits in juices and smoothies helps to increase the number of servings of fresh fruits and vegetables in your daily diet.

The best way to make sure you're getting the vitamins and minerals you need is by drinking the rainbow. Fruits and vegetables come in a rainbow of colors — red, orange, yellow, green, blue, indigo, and violet — and it's easy to get optimum nutrients from the food you eat by including one or more foods in each color every day. Here are examples of places where you can get all the colors of the rainbow:

- ✔ **Red:** Beets, cherries, cranberries, pink grapefruit, pomegranates, raspberries, red cabbage, red grapes, red peppers, red potatoes, rhubarb, strawberries, tomatoes, watermelon

- ✔ **Orange:** Apricots, cantaloupe, carrots, mangoes, nectarines, orange peppers, papayas, persimmons, pumpkins, squash, sweet potatoes

✔ **Yellow:** Citrus fruit, corn, grapefruit, peaches, pears, pineapple, rutabaga, yellow peppers, yellow summer squash, yellow tomatoes, yellow watermelon

✔ **Green:** Asparagus, avocadoes, beet greens, broccoli, Brussels sprouts, collard greens, cucumbers, green beans, green cabbage, green grapes, green peppers, honeydew melon, kale, kiwi, limes, mustard greens, peas, spinach, Swiss chard, turnip greens, zucchini

✔ **Blue:** Blueberries, concord grapes

✔ **Indigo:** Blackberries, dates, elderberries, figs, plums, prunes, raisins

✔ **Violet:** Eggplant, plums, purple grapes

✔ **White:** Bananas, cauliflower, garlic, ginger, jicama, mushrooms, onions, parsnips, potatoes, turnips

Chapter 6

Juices and Smoothies for the Outside

In This Chapter

▶ Looking younger, feeling better

▶ Improving your skin

▶ Building healthy hair and nails

▶ Shedding extra pounds

*B*eauty is more than skin deep. In fact, it reaches right down to the molecules and cells of your body. Organs and blood, bone and flesh — vibrant good looks radiate outward from them. When all the body's systems, especially the organs of elimination and digestion, are working at their best, it's reflected in your skin, eyes, nails, and hair. You glow with a clean and honest beauty that has nothing to do with perfect features, artful makeup, or the right clothes.

Vibrant, healthy good looks are your natural reward from what you choose to eat and drink and the exercise you get on a daily basis. In this chapter, I call on science to explain the factors that contribute to aging so that you can understand how consuming fresh fruits and vegetables actually saves your body from the ravages of time.

Glowing skin, bright eyes, shining hair, and strong nails are the other benefits of smoothies and juices that I explore. Are you hoping to lose weight? This chapter helps you to achieve optimum health and weight by taking you through the practical steps you need to take in order to achieve realistic goals.

Looking your best on the outside may spur you to learn more about juicing and blending for the inside. It's all connected; keep reading to Chapter 7.

Looking Younger

Everyone knows what happens in aging — the loss of strength and energy, the slowing of the mental processes and memory, the graying hair, and changes to the skeleton and skin — but do you understand what aging actually *is?* Here are a couple of things to consider before you submit to the general theory that you can't win the fight against aging:

- From about the time you reach puberty, you begin to age. Aging is a continuous process that can be slowed but not stopped. Why not concentrate on slowing the process, protecting the cells against damage, and staying healthy longer?

- Aging is a progressive process that worsens with time, accumulating and compounding. Why not protect the immune system so that the body isn't weakened, and so that cells are strong and the domino effect of cell destruction is not allowed to open the door to fatal diseases?

Maybe you can't win, but you can definitely score some points and enjoy the game.

What exactly is aging? It could be that the body is designed to age and there is a biological timeline that our bodies follow. Or maybe changes in hormones control aging. Or maybe the immune system is programmed to decline over time, leaving people more susceptible to diseases. Other aging theories assert that, like electronic products and car engines, cells and tissues simply wear out. Others reason that the faster an organism uses oxygen, the shorter it lives. All these theories may contribute in a large or small part to aging.

Science has proved that molecules known as *free radicals* cause damage to cells, and this destruction leaves them vulnerable to disease and premature aging.

There is no doubt that your body is continually undergoing complex biochemical functions, reactions, and changes and that time is exacting a toll. The one thing that you can do to counteract them and protect the cells, the immune system, and other vital organs is to feed them the high-quality nutrients they need to stay toxin-free and functioning at optimal levels.

Juices and smoothies allow you to absorb the nutrients from fruits and vegetables. This is important because, as you age, your digestive function diminishes or is impaired by toxins or years of poor food choices. The nutrients in juices and smoothies pass directly into your blood because they've been broken down, or "pre-digested," so that they don't put any strain on your digestive system.

Vitamin C is necessary for the synthesis of collagen, which in turn keeps all your tissues (including your skin) in tip-top condition. Vitamin A found in the deep red, orange, and green fruits and vegetables is converted to retinol by the body. Retinol protects the surface of the eye, or the *cornea,* and is essential for good vision. And it just so happens that the fruits and vegetables high in vitamins C and A are also high in antioxidants.

Focusing on free radical damage

Free radicals are highly unstable molecules that are dangerous because they lack an electron, which causes them to latch on to other molecules in the body in order to steal an electron from them. In doing this, free radicals damage vital cell structures, thus destroying DNA, enzymes, proteins, and membranes and causing them to malfunction. Free radicals are a product of stress, chemical pollutants, and toxins, as well as normal cell function. When cells create energy by metabolizing food or when our immune systems attack microorganisms, these essential cell activities produce unstable oxygen molecules known as *free radicals.*

There is no escaping the fact that your body will be producing the very agents of aging that contribute to wrinkles, sagging skin, loss of muscle tone, age spots, and the onset of age-related diseases. But there is a powerful tool that your body can use to mop up free radicals and prevent them from doing harm. That important preventive tool is the group of nutrients known as *antioxidants.*

Antioxidants are substances found in plants that act as sponges in your body to soak up free radicals. There has been a tremendous amount of research surrounding antioxidant vitamins (vitamins A, C, and E) and their role in slowing aging, boosting immune response, and reducing the risk of degenerative diseases.

If the foods you eat provide plenty of high-quality antioxidants, they can neutralize free radical damage and slow aging. Antioxidants are found in bright and dark red, orange, or green plant foods. (See Chapter 20 for a list of ten antioxidant-rich fruits and vegetables.)

Making smoothies and juices from enzyme- and antioxidant-rich fruits and vegetables means that you're releasing these virtual sponges into your body. Antioxidants and enzymes work together on the inside of cells to protect against free radicals, and antioxidants also circulate through the blood to neutralize free radicals outside the cell structures.

Preventing or reversing age spots

Often called "liver spots," these flat brown areas may begin to appear on the face, hands, arms, legs, chest, and neck around middle age (thus, the term *age spots*). Age spots are a result of exposure to the sun. Over time, our skin is subjected to increasing amounts of sun damage to the *melanocytes* (skin cells that produce melanin pigment, which helps to protect us from the sun).

In fact, age spots have nothing to do with how old you are. Instead, they're related to how long you've been exposed to the sun and how good a job your melanocytes work. Fair-skinned people tend to have more of these dark spots than their dark-skinned counterparts.

Free radical damage (in this case, from the sun) is at the root of the problem. When you see dark spots on your skin, they're an indication that the cells are damaged and are accumulating waste.

Again, foods high in antioxidants can protect skin cells from free radical destruction. In addition, one to three days of juice fasting helps to cleanse your body at the cellular level because your body can concentrate on cleanup and repair when it doesn't have to use its resources for digestion. A juice fast is an opportunity for your body to clean out the wastes that have accumulated, including those that are clumped together on the top layers of your skin. (See Chapter 10 for more on fasting and detoxing.)

Using a mineral sunscreen, such as zinc or titanium, early in life will help to prevent formation of age spots.

If you notice a new bump or dark spot on your skin, or if a spot you've had for a while starts to change, consult a doctor to make sure it's not cancerous.

Recognizing the anti-aging, restorative power of green juices

Like the green foods they're made from, green juices are bursting with chlorophyll, enzymes, and phytonutrients, in a combination that's perfect for rebuilding, rejuvenating, and regenerating cells; energizing the body; protecting cells from free radicals, radiation, and degenerative diseases; as well as boosting immune performance. All this prevention and restorative power makes them powerful anti-aging drinks.

Table 6-1 lists green ingredients and the nutrients they contain.

Table 6-1	The Nutrients in Green Foods	
Food	*What It Offers the Body*	*What It Can Help*
Alfalfa sprouts	Calcium, chlorine, magnesium, phosphorus, potassium, silicon, sodium, zinc; vitamins A, B complex, C, E, and K; amino acids; and chlorophyll	Anemia, eye problems, fatigue, hair loss, liver and kidney disorders, thyroid gland regulation, weight loss
Artichokes (mixed with other juices to alleviate the starchy taste)	Non-starchy carbohydrates and insulin	Reduces sweet cravings; may be helpful for diabetics, hypoglycemia, and weight loss
Asparagus	Vitamins A, B1, B9, and C; potassium; choline	Reduces acidity in blood; cleanses tissues and muscles; helps dissolve kidney stones
Bean sprouts (aduki, mung, lentils, and other dried beans)	Protein; iron; vitamin C	Builds blood; the presence of vitamin C helps the body absorb more iron; helps prevent anemia, arthritis, cancer; reduces fluid, fatigue; aids in weight loss
Cabbage, broccoli, cauliflower, daikon, Brussels sprouts, collard greens, horse-radish, kale, kohlrabi, mustard greens, radish, rutabaga, turnip root and greens, watercress, wasabi	Vitamins A, B6, and C; calcium, chlorine, iodine, potassium, sulfur	Tonic and cleanser; ulcer healing; kidney problems; skin disorders; yeast infections; helps prevent cancer; lowers cholesterol
Dandelion greens	Vitamins A, B1, and C; calcium, iron, potassium, sodium, magnesium	Tonic and cleanser, especially the liver; blood alkalizer; improves night blindness; acne; anemia; kidney, liver disorders; weight loss

(continued)

Table 6-1 *(continued)*

Food	What It Offers the Body	What It Can Help
Cabbage, broccoli, cauliflower, daikon, Brussels sprouts, collard greens, horseradish, kale, kohlrabi, mustard greens, radish, rutabaga, turnip root and greens, watercress, wasabi, lettuce, spinach, Swiss chard	Calcium, iron, magnesium, potassium; vitamins A and E; chlorophyll	Anemia, constipation, liver and kidney disorders, nerves, stimulates circulation, weight loss
Wheatgrass, sprouted wheat berries	Vitamins A, B complex, C, and E; full spectrum of minerals and trace elements	Cleansing, restorative, rejuvenating, protects the heart, anemia, arthritis, asthma, bladder problems, cancer, eye problems, liver and kidney disorders, ulcers, weight loss

Other green ingredients include celery, cucumber, endive, fennel, fenugreek, broccoli, sunflower sprouts, lamb's quarters, herbs (especially parsley), and sweet bell peppers.

Start slowly and add highly potent green ingredients to juice ingredients, slowly building the amounts, but never adding more than one-quarter greens to three-quarters other vegetables.

Recharging your batteries

An active person's *metabolic rate* (the amount of energy you burn while at rest) burns hotter and faster than that of an inactive person. Increasing activity requires the body to burn more calories, which come from excess body fat or from the food you consume.

The benefits of increasing your activity level are that your body weight will drop, and you'll be providing your body with a wider variety of vitamins and minerals (including antioxidant or anti-aging nutrients) because of the extra food you'll be consuming to fuel your exercise. In addition, your body will get better at using the vitamins and minerals it takes in, and this results in healthier cells, thus slowing the aging process.

Acne busters

When pores and hair follicles become blocked, *sebum*, the skin's natural oil, can't drain and bacteria infect it, causing blackheads and whiteheads to form just under the skin. Fasting can help to clear the cells of waste. Cleansing the skin on the outside with gentle facial soap and cleansing it on the inside is the very best remedy for acne that you'll ever find.

In addition, diet is important to reducing inflammation and keeping the skin follicles open and clear. Foods for your face that are rich in vitamins A, B complex, and C and smoothies and juices that are made from melons, spinach, and other dark leafy greens (parsley, kale, and Swiss chard) and broccoli can help treat acne. Yellow-orange vegetables and fruits, for example, apricots, red peppers, carrots, squash, and carrots are bursting with anti-inflammatory beta carotene, another good acne buster.

Fruit smoothies and juices provide the best energy for recharging your batteries if you're an active person. For an excellent energy juice, try juicing the following:

- 1 apple
- 1 slice pineapple
- 1 slice watermelon or cantaloupe
- 2 carrots
- 1 wedge of cabbage

Combine the following ingredients in the blender for an energy smoothie:

- ½ cup orange juice
- ¼ cup carrot juice
- 1 cup watermelon cubes or seedless grapes
- 1 cup cantaloupe cubes
- ½ cup fresh or frozen berries

Improving Your Skin

The transformation of your skin to a flawless, glowing complexion starts on the inside. Nutrients and pure water found in raw fruits and vegetables are the keys to beautiful skin, and drinking pure fruit and vegetable juices or smoothies feeds and enables the growth of healthy skin cells that will transform your skin.

Your body's skin is actually one of the biggest organs, and it's made up of several layers. The outer layer, or *epidermis,* acts as a barrier to environmental damage from bacteria and toxic chemicals, as well as from the sun's rays, and it assists in the elimination of toxins from the body. The *dermis* cells (the deeper layers of the skin) nourish the epidermis and replenish the cells of the epidermis and its millions of dead cells on the surface that are constantly being shed. This is the layer that is made from elastin and collagen that forms the structure of your skin. It gives firmness to the skin and can sag or become creased with lines. Overexposure to sun damages the dermis, making it leathery and wrinkled. The deepest layer of skin is called the *hypodermis;* this is where sweat glands, hair follicles, and main blood vessels of the skin are found.

A layer of dead cells that have undergone a process called *keratinization* forms the top layer of the epidermis. This top layer has had the protein hardened. That's what makes the top skin cells waterproof.

Vitamin C improves the suppleness of the skin because it builds collagen. Collagen is made up of proteins that form the "glue" used by the body to connect and support tissues such as skin, bone, tendons, muscles, organs, teeth, gums, and cartilage. Fruits and vegetables high in vitamin C — citrus fruit, strawberries, cabbage, and peppers — are essential for healthy skin.

In addition to vitamin C, a host of nutrients found in fruits and vegetables are essential to healthy skin. Vitamin A helps the skin rid itself of blemishes and stimulates the renewal of skin cells; vitamin E protects against skin cancer, speeds healing of cuts and abrasions, and prevents dryness; calcium

Cleansing your body to improve your skin

Results from a two- to three-day fruit cleanse vary, but you'll notice a visible difference in the texture, firmness, and contour of your skin, which should lead to a lessening in the number and depth of facial lines and wrinkles. The skin (as well as your hair and eyes) will exhibit a bright, clear glow.

It's best to juice-cleanse over a weekend, starting and finishing with raw foods on the days just before and after you're actually only drinking pure water along with fresh, raw fruit juices. You can sip as many juices as you want during the fast, depending on how hungry you get, but six is the usual number to expect to drink each day. (See Chapter 10 for more details.)

supports the bones so that skin doesn't sag or wrinkle; and essential fatty acids feed the skin, making it soft and plump instead of dry and lined.

 Water is essential for healthy cells, including skin cells. Regular water intake in the form of pure water or the fluids in fruits and vegetables helps to flush waste that causes dull, lifeless skin. Because fruits and vegetables are over 90 percent pure water that has been naturally filtered through the plant's root system, they're an excellent way to hydrate the cells of your body.

Growing Healthy Hair and Nails

What is one of the easiest ways for nutritionists and other health professionals to determine malnourishment, nutrient minerals, and trace elements your body may be lacking, and even toxic exposure to elements like lead, cadmium, mercury, aluminum, or arsenic? By analyzing your hair. That's because hair permanently records your body's levels of these important nutrients and offers a snapshot of your body's state at a particular time.

The reason hair analysis is so accurate and reliable is that when new hair cells are forming the hair follicle, they take in traces of substances in the blood stream — protein, fat, vitamins, minerals, and trace elements, as well as toxic substances. New cells push out the older cells, and as the hair or nail cells move away from the follicle or nail bed, they die and harden, trapping and mapping exactly what was in them or lacking in them at the time of the cells' death.

Healthy hair and nails have a natural luster, strength, and shine that come directly from the nutrients in the blood vessels in the dermis at the base of the hair follicle and the nail bed. Feeding the cells that are important for the regenerative growth of both hair and nails means that when they eventually die and are keratinized, they will be stronger.

Sebum, the body's natural oil, comes from the sebaceous gland connected to the hair follicle. When the oil is replenished from the foods you eat and drink, it coats the hair and gives it more luster and natural shine.

You already know that juicing and smoothies will deliver concentrated vitamins and minerals, as well as some protein, carbohydrate, and fat, depending on the ingredients you choose to add. And you know that those nutrients pass directly into your blood from fruit and vegetable juices because the fiber has been removed. Table 6-2 lists the specific foods to juice daily or add to your smoothies to feed your hair and nails.

Table 6-2	Nutrients for Strong Hair and Nails	
Nutrient	**How It Helps Hair and Nails**	**What Foods to Juice or Blend**
Protein	A protein known as *keratin* strengthens hair and nails, so protein provides the structure for growing strong hair and nails.	Low-fat dairy (yogurt, milk), nuts, soymilk, sea vegetables (for smoothies)
Omega-3 fatty acids	Help form healthy sebum and support scalp health, keeping it from drying and flaking.	Chia seeds, flaxseed, fish oil, seafood, walnuts
Vitamin A	Keeps the root and bulb of hair follicles healthy, helps produce sebum, actually helps increase hair growth.	Apricots, broccoli, cantaloupe, carrots, mangoes, spinach, squash, kale, parsley, chard, beet greens, sweet peppers
B-complex vitamins	Prevent hair loss and graying hair; strengthen nails.	Dark green, leafy vegetables; oats, nuts and legumes.
Vitamin D	The presence of vitamin D receptor cells on the hair indicates that it regulates rate of hair growth.	Greek yogurt, milk, sunflower sprouts
Biotin	Improves splitting or thinning hair and strengthens nails. Deficiency can cause hair loss.	Bananas, legumes, brewer's yeast, soy products, pecans, walnuts, peanuts, and oatmeal (all added to smoothies)
Copper	Deficiency may result in white, silver, or gray hair color and thin, lifeless hair.	Carrots, garlic, ginger, turnips, papaya, and apples
Zinc	Important to the formation of connective tissue. White spots on nails, hair loss, hair dryness, and brittleness are signs of zinc deficiency.	Ginger, parsley, garlic, carrots, grapes, spinach, cabbage, cucumbers, green beans, soybeans

Losing Weight

A few years ago, I lost 30 pounds over the course of a year. I was pleased that I had accomplished my goal and that, in the process, I didn't actually feel like I had deprived myself of good food. What surprised me the most about the reaction of my friends and family was their one question: "How did you lose weight?"

I'm here to tell you what I told them: There is no magic involved in losing weight. Anyone who makes a commitment to being healthy and losing weight can do it. There is only one sure route to weight loss, and that is to make sure that you burn more calories than you take in.

Your body converts what you eat and drink into energy using a process called *metabolism*. Calories from protein, carbohydrate, or fat are combined with oxygen during this complex biochemical process to release the energy your body needs to work and move and even for internal functions while you're sleeping or at rest.

The number of calories your body uses to satisfy its energy needs is called your basal metabolic rate (BMR). It's based on your age, sex, and body size and composition. Your BMR should account for 60 percent to 75 percent of the calories you burn every day. BMR is the number of calories that nutritionists use to calculate how many calories you should be eating in a day to lose or gain weight.

The only factor that can change the number of calories your body burns or converts to energy in a day is physical activity.

If you eat or drink fewer calories than your body burns over the course of time, it will begin to use energy stored as fat to fuel its BMR and physical activity. If you want to lose weight and you choose not to increase the amount of physical activity you do in a day, you'll have to decrease the number of calories you consume. If you change to lower-fat foods and decrease the number of calories you take in *and* you begin to add some form of physical activity to your daily routine, you'll burn fat and lose weight at a faster rate.

Taking the long-term approach

Remember I mentioned that I took a year to lose 30 pounds? That works out to about 2½ pounds per month. Not all that impressive when stacked up against the claims of some popular diets, I admit. However, slow, steady

The role of fat in weight gain or loss

Of all the nutrients in food, only proteins, carbohydrates, and fats contain calories. And fat contains over two times the number of calories per gram that proteins or carbohydrates contain.

You need complex carbohydrates like those found in fruits and vegetables; lean protein from nuts, beans, soy, chicken, and fish; and small amounts (not more than 25 percent of your total calories) of polyunsaturated fats like avocado oil, olive oil, and nut oils. The focus should be on omega-3 fats because they're the types of fats least consumed in the modern Western diet.

Because fat is over twice as concentrated in calories as protein or carbohydrates and because it enters the body in a state ready to be stored, consumption of high-fat foods in amounts not balanced by physical activity leads to weight gain, so use it sparingly. It's important to note that excess carbohydrates are easily converted and stored as fat if they aren't used by the body for energy.

One of the most important advantages of pure fruit or vegetable juices and smoothies is that, while they contain plant proteins and carbohydrates, they're completely free of fat. This makes them valuable snack and meal substitutes to use as part of your new, healthy routine.

weight loss has proven to be the most effective method of keeping you motivated and of being able to maintain your new, healthy weight.

You stay motivated by taking a long-term approach because losing one to six pounds a month means that you're setting reasonable goals instead of starving or depriving yourself only to go right back to old habits when the diet is finished. It gives you results you can track, and it means that you're revamping your eating habits over a longer period of time and training yourself to rethink your attitudes about food, health, and weight.

To lose 1 pound of fat, a person must consume or burn (through exercise) 3,500 calories less than he or she uses.

Making lifestyle changes

In addition to reducing calories in and increasing calories out, there are other factors that guarantee success in achieving and maintaining an appropriate weight. Having a positive attitude and making a commitment based on reasonable goals will ensure long-term success in your weight loss program. Here are some of the adjustments that will prove to be the most important changes you'll ever make because they take you away from crash or temporary diet toward permanent lifestyle changes:

- **Eat and drink low-fat foods.** Juices and smoothies are excellent low-fat meal replacement and snack alternatives. Every individual's caloric needs varies, but generally, a successful weight-loss program provides 1,200 to 1,500 calories per day. Eating complex carbohydrates in the form of raw fruits and vegetables will give you a feeling of being full with over half the calories of a high-fat meal.

  Eating large amounts of high-fat foods promotes weight gain and keeps fat stored on the body.

- **Increase fiber.** Drinking fruit or vegetable smoothies helps increase your fiber intake. Insoluble and soluble fiber are found only in plant foods. Fiber is most abundant in fresh raw fruits and vegetables. The *bulk* from fruits and vegetables is due to the fiber and cellulose in plant foods, which gives a feeling of fullness and means that you'll stop eating sooner. Raw fruits and vegetables contain no fat and are relatively low in calories and provide consistent energy production.

  Metabolizing stored fat during weight loss releases toxins in those cells, and fiber helps eliminate those wastes.

  Mix 1 tablespoon of psyllium husk powder into fresh juices or smoothies and take before and between meals to help reduce appetite. Be sure to drink eight glasses of water daily.

- **Drink fresh juices and smoothies every day.** For snacks between meals, juices are best because they provide pure absorbable nutrients quickly. A great start to any weight-loss program is to begin with a one- to three-day juice fast. Drink fresh fruit juice at breakfast and midmorning and take fresh vegetable juices after that, for lunch, midafternoon, at dinner-time, and midevening. This feeds your body an abundance of absorbable nutrients while allowing your stomach muscles to relax and contract. (See Chapter 10 for details on cleansing with juice.)

- **Use smoothies for meal replacements.** Smoothies are excellent because the fiber in them gives a feeling of fullness that stays with you longer. Substitute all high-fat, empty-calorie snacks with fresh juice and replace one meal with a smoothie, and you'll reduce your overall calorie intake dramatically.

  Consider enjoying a one-day juice fast every week to keep flushing the body with pure, absorbable nutrients, which help to reduce cravings.

✔ **Drink eight glasses of pure water every day.** Pure water is essential, and you can count pure juice or herbal teas as one or two of the eight recommended glasses. Every time you crave something or feel hungry, drink a glass of water (or juice or smoothie, depending on the time of day and convenience) because it will give you a feeling of fullness. Water hydrates your cells, suppresses your appetite, and works with the extra fiber from raw fruits and vegetables to flush toxins and metabolize fat from the body.

✔ **Eliminate sugar and sweet beverages and foods.** Never use artificial sweeteners. Natural and refined sugars are mostly empty calories, meaning that they offer no nutrients and are more likely to get stored as fat than used for energy by your body. Sweets stimulate the appetite so, strictly speaking, all-fruit juices or smoothies should be avoided when you're in a weight-loss program, unless you're using them in a cleanse.

Artificial sweeteners stimulate the appetite and add to toxic waste in the cells.

✔ **Exercise regularly.** Walk, run, jog, practice yoga, dance, cycle, swim, play tennis, or engage in another sport as part of your exercise program. Our bodies are made to move, and when they don't get the activity they were designed for, they begin to store excess energy as fat. Exercise is essential for weight loss and for healthy, fit bodies.

Find a way to include at least 30 minutes of moderate activity or exercise four to five times per week.

✔ **Choose healthy foods all the time.** Eating six small portions of whole foods and one or two juices or smoothies is healthier than three large, high-fat meals.

The reason I call these suggestions healthy lifestyle habits is that, in order for you to see permanent results in fitness, health, and weight, you need to make permanent changes to your attitude about food and the food choices you make from here on out. This is not a diet to endure and then slip back to the old ways. Changing the habit of what you have for meals and snacks is the key to achieving and maintaining a healthy weight.

Healthy foods include small amounts of lean sources of protein — nuts, whole grains, legumes, fish, lean dairy, lean meats — with eight to ten servings of fresh fruits and vegetables.

The good news is that with the help of a juice cleanse and regular intake of juices and smoothies, cravings, especially sweet cravings, will stop within the first few days and your appetite for fat will decrease. As your body is nourished by the whole foods you eat and drink, the body will be less stressed and working at its optimum, and digestion will be working properly. You'll find that your energy levels rise with exercise and healthy eating habits.

Staying regular with fruit and fiber

Eating fiber is one of the easiest and least expensive ways to prevent disease and maintain health and a reasonable weight because it helps the body to eliminate waste materials and deadly toxins. Unlike soluble fiber, which absorbs water to form a gel and which pushes food along the digestive tract, insoluble fiber doesn't dissolve, so it moves through the intestines virtually intact and without being absorbed.

Insoluble fiber, found in apple skins, cherries, grapes, pineapple, rhubarb, oranges, melons, dates, prunes, and berries, adds bulk to stomach and bowel movements, reducing constipation and causing you to feel full, thus helping with appetite control. Vegetables high in insoluble fiber include turnips, beets, cauliflower, cabbage, Brussels sprouts, and carrots. Fruits and vegetables are best if eaten raw because cooking softens the fiber and breaks down some of the cellular structure.

Snacking on juices and smoothies

Do you find yourself eating in your car, in front of the computer or television, or while in the kitchen, preparing dinner? Those are the worst times to snack because they're mindless consumption, not usually because you're actually hungry, and the choices are usually empty-calorie, high-salt, high-fat foods.

Do you drink several cups or glasses of carbonated drinks, iced tea, coffee, or flavored water? Next time you reach for your favorite drink, check the number of calories in it and multiply them by the average number of times you drink them in a day. Drinking sugar, caffeine, artificial sugar, and calories is an unconscious habit that can be easily eliminated.

Choosing a juice or smoothie as a snack does two things:

✔ It causes you to think about what you're doing and signals that you have actually chosen to include this food in your daily routine instead of absently munching.

✔ It actually helps to reduce cravings and quenches thirst because it provides pure water and nutrients directly to the blood stream.

Vegetables are the best choice for juice and smoothie snacks when weight loss is a goal.

Drinking juices and smoothies as meal replacements

Before you start to think that I'm recommending that you use juices and smoothies as a substitute for a balanced diet, let me be clear: They should always be an *integrated part of* a balanced diet. Having said that, you can start to control the amount of calories and the portions of foods you consume within a balanced diet by drinking a juice or smoothie for one meal in your day on an occasional basis.

Keeping a food log and knowing the total calories you consume each day is a pretty good exercise for anyone serious about losing weight. It not only shows you how much you consume, but also helps to pinpoint the high-calorie foods. A successful weight-loss program provides 1,200 to 1,500 calories per day. You can divide your day into five light meals and three light snacks, allowing roughly 200 calories per meal and between 100 and 150 calories for the snacks. If you're still eating three main meals and one or two snacks in a day, that works out to roughly 350 to 400 calories per meal and 100 to 200 calories for the snacks. It's important for you to get an idea of how many calories are in the foods you eat every day and how to keep everything you eat — meals, drinks, and snacks — in line with a reasonable calorie goal for your age, sex, and physical activity.

Drinking a pure vegetable juice or smoothie is an excellent way to nourish your body with vitamins, minerals, and phytonutrients, while lowering calories because they're are virtually fat-free and lower in natural sugars than fruit. Here are some tips for making juices and smoothies to replace a meal:

- ✔ **Choose mostly vegetables and use fruit sparingly.** One apple or other fruit to three vegetables is a good ratio to follow for juices or smoothies.

- ✔ **Use only low-fat dairy products in smoothies.** Skip cheese and ice cream and check labels on yogurt for artificial sweeteners and other ingredients used as thickeners; use skim or 1 percent milk in smoothies.

- ✔ **Use only your own juices in smoothies.** Juicing your own apples or oranges for the liquid in smoothies will reduce the calories significantly because bottled juices tend to be higher in calories.

- ✔ **Add some protein.** Stir a tablespoon of flaxseeds, chia seeds, nuts, tofu, or whey powder into juice or smoothies.

- ✔ **Include dark greens.** Adding kale, Swiss chard, spinach, or broccoli boosts calcium.

- ✔ **Avoid dried and canned fruit.** They're usually high in sugar, and some are treated with chemicals.

Flushing fats with juice, water, and smoothies

Your digestive system, especially your liver, is important to maintaining overall health and, specifically, to maintaining optimal body weight. That's because the liver is the primary organ for filtering out pollutants and chemicals from your food and, just as important, metabolizes fat. Detoxifying and cleansing the liver makes it more efficient so that nutrients are absorbed, waste and toxins are cleared, and fat is burned more effectively.

Eating organic foods and avoiding over-the-counter drugs as much as possible is the first step in helping the liver do its job. The next is to drink those eight glasses of water! Last, cleansing the liver is absolutely essential.

A juice fast to cleanse the liver and lymphatic system is one of the keys to your health. I guarantee you'll feel better, and it'll help your liver work with you as you begin to lose weight. Here is a simple plan for a liver cleanse:

- ✔ **Day 1: Pre-cleanse:** Eat only raw foods — no dairy, no grains, no animal protein. Here are some suggestions:

    - Make a fresh, raw fruit juice for breakfast and a midmorning snack (see Chapter 12 for recipes, but omit all dairy).

    - Either eat ten raw almonds throughout the day or grind them and stir half of them into your breakfast and midmorning juices.

    - Make a fresh green salad for lunch and dress it with 2 tablespoons of organic, cold-pressed nut, avocado, or olive oil mixed with 3 tablespoons of apple cider vinegar.

    - In the midafternoon, make a fresh, raw vegetable juice with a beet and some greens — you can pick a vegetable juice recipe from Chapter 12 and add the beet and greens, or use the Borscht recipe in Chapter 12 and omit the yogurt.

    - For dinner, either eat a fresh vegetable salad or drink a vegetable smoothie. In the mid-evening, drink a vegetable smoothie.

    - Be sure to drink eight glasses of pure water throughout the day. You can have herbal tea, but no coffee or black tea.

- ✔ **Days 2, 3, and (optional) 4: Cleanse:** Drink only pure juice or water. Here are some suggestions:

    - Upon rising, drink a glass of fresh pure water mixed with the juice of ½ lemon. Wait an hour, and make a fresh, raw fruit juice as your breakfast.

- Juice 4 cups fresh cranberries and 1 apple; measure the juice and add an equal amount of pure water. Cover and set aside in the refrigerator. Drink 1 cup midmorning and 1 cup midafternoon.

- At noon, drink a vegetable juice and drink a vegetable juice again every two hours after that.

- Be sure to drink eight glasses of pure water throughout the day. You can have herbal tea, but no coffee or black tea.

✔ **Day 4 or 5: Post-cleanse:** Eat only raw foods — no dairy, no grains, no animal protein. Here are some suggestions:

- Make a fresh, raw fruit juice for breakfast and a midmorning snack (see Chapter 12 for recipes, but omit all dairy).

- Either eat ten raw almonds throughout the day or grind them and stir half of them into your breakfast and midmorning juices.

- Make a fresh green salad for lunch and dress it with 2 tablespoons of organic, cold-pressed nut, avocado, or olive oil mixed with 3 tablespoons of apple cider vinegar.

- In the midafternoon, make a fresh, raw vegetable juice with a beet and some greens — you can pick a vegetable juice recipe from Chapter 12 and add the beet and greens, or use the Borscht recipe in Chapter 12 and omit the yogurt.

- For dinner, either eat a fresh vegetable salad or drink a vegetable smoothie. In the mid-evening, drink a vegetable smoothie.

- Be sure to drink eight glasses of pure water throughout the day. You can have herbal tea, but no coffee or black tea.

Chapter 7

Juices and Smoothies for the Inside

In This Chapter

▶ Feeling energized and sexy

▶ Improving immunity and memory

Given that modern society is fast-paced and stress-filled with escalating demands on your time and patience and seemingly little choice for nourishing food, it's not surprising that many people consider wellness and health to be the absence of sickness and disease. But high-level wellness — that clear-headed, exuberant, and joyful state of being that encompasses social, mental, emotional, and physical fitness and well-being — involves so much more than simply not being sick.

Emerging from the fog of low-level nutrition in order to be vibrant and clearly alive is something that is possible for everyone to achieve through diet and exercise. It's not by chance that some people are lean and strong and resistant to illness, have sharp brains, and stay sexually vibrant.

Instead, it's the small day-to-day decisions that revolve around conscious and unconscious habits that raise or lower your own level of health. This chapter is all about feeding your body at a cellular level so that each intricate component can fulfill its brilliant potential and compose the shining entity that you are. It's about bringing on physical and mental change from the inside.

Increasing Your Energy Level

People are meant to think and move, dance and play. They're wired for contemplation, recollection, memory, and throwing their entire beings into their passions. And at the end of the day, they may be spent and tired and ready for a long, rejuvenating sleep, but they've also been able to think clearly and act with vitality. They feel rewarded for their efforts and their ability to handle whatever the day has presented. Operating at a low, depressed, irritable, and lethargic pace is crippling in an insidious way — but it's often a normal way of life for people who think they don't have time to eat well, replenish their spirits, and exercise.

Ironically, people who take the time to nourish their bodies and spirits and who set aside a mere 30 minutes for physical activity every day actually have more time for all the daily routine tasks, as well as the unplanned challenges, because they're mentally, emotionally, and physically equipped to accomplish their goals and handle the stresses, which allows them to get more done. Increasing your energy level through cleansing and flushing (see Chapter 10) and feeding and fueling the cells not only infuses your body, but also begins to change your thinking and your emotions in ways that you may not expect.

In their raw state, all plants (in particular, fruits) are reservoirs of solar energy. The presence of this incredible energy is what makes raw plant food so vital to your health. It's what separates synthesized chemical supplements from the vitamins, minerals, and other nutrients in the real thing. Fresh, raw fruit is higher in solar energy than any other plant, although vegetables, grains, nuts, seeds, and legumes all contribute that life-giving force if you eat them raw. Food plants that have a long, slow ripening process and that are ripened on the vine or in the field (instead of in gas-filled containers or on shelves) have more time to absorb and store the sun's energy, and that's why most fruits are exceptional energy storehouses. Naturally sun-dried fruit or vegetables are also high in solar energy.

The sun's energy is stored in the cells of plants as starch. Starch is one of the body's primary sources of complex carbohydrates, and starch is converted to glycogen (sugar), which is pure energy in your body. It's this carbohydrate-to-sugar-to-energy process (called *metabolism*) within human beings that powers everything you do. It fuels your growth, allows you to breathe and carry on all the daily and nightly involuntary internal functions, and allows you to think and be active.

Fueling the body

In order to capture and utilize a high level of dynamism and drive, you need to provide your body with energy. Foods high in complex carbohydrates and high-quality whole foods, as well as omega-3 fatty acids, are healthy energy foods. Here's how they work:

✔ **Complex carbohydrates:** These essential macronutrients are converted to glucose and are either used immediately for energy or additional glucose is turned into glycogen and stored in the muscles and liver for energy at a later time. As opposed to simple carbohydrates (found in white sugar and processed grain products), complex carbohydrates are bound up in soluble and insoluble fiber, so they take longer for the body to digest. This means that they supply a slower, steady source of energy resulting in stamina and endurance.

Juice a wide variety of fresh fruits and vegetables, and eat whole grains, legumes, nuts, and seeds to get plenty of complex carbohydrates.

✔ **B vitamins:** B vitamins are essential for proper metabolism, and B6 works with enzymes to convert carbohydrates to glycogen. Without the B vitamins, energy from food wouldn't be as efficiently used. A deficiency over time results in extreme fatigue and reduced resistance to allergies and infection.

To get enough B vitamins, juice green leafy vegetables, broccoli, cauliflower, and kale. Eat whole grains, poultry, fish, eggs, nuts, beans, and lean meats.

✔ **Potassium:** Potassium carries a slight positive electrical charge and plays a key role in energy metabolism in the body. Deficiency is associated with muscle weakness, confusion, chronic fatigue, and exhaustion.

To get enough potassium, juice a wide variety of fruits and vegetables; the best sources include Swiss chard, spinach, papaya, parsley, garlic, broccoli, cauliflower, watercress, asparagus, red cabbage, cantaloupes, tomatoes, beets, and peaches. Also, eat potatoes, legumes, and lentils.

✔ **Antioxidants:** The natural process of metabolizing food to energy releases free radicals, which can damage cells. Antioxidants neutralize free radicals.

To get plenty of antioxidants, juice brightly colored fruit and vegetables, and eat whole grains and nuts.

✔ **Proteins:** Protein forms the building blocks for cells, tissues, muscles, bones, cartilage, and skin. Muscle burns energy at a faster rate than fat cells do, so using protein to build muscle is important in weight loss.

Add ground nuts and seeds and cooked lentils to smoothies and juices to get plenty of protein.

✔ **Essential fatty acids:** Keep your cells and brain functioning properly with essential fatty acids. A lack of essential fatty acids can disrupt the balance of energy in your body by preventing your brain and cells from performing at their peak.

Add ground nuts and seeds and cooked lentils to smoothies and juices to get enough essential fatty acids.

Building bones

Your skeleton supports you and enables you to be physical, so keeping your bones in top condition is important to your ability to be active and energetic. Although calcium is a critical bone-building mineral, other nutrients play a key role in keeping your bones strong and healthy, too. Getting plenty of fruits and vegetables by drinking juices or smoothies leads to greater bone density.

For example, high levels of magnesium are linked to strong bones and calcium retention; omega-3 fatty acids decrease the rate of bone breakdown and facilitate consistent bone formation; vitamin K is critical in forming bone proteins and reduces the risk of hip fractures; vitamin D assists in calcium absorption. In addition, weight-bearing exercises like running, dancing, and lifting weights stress your bones and keep their cells regenerating.

For healthy bones, juice dark green leafy vegetables, broccoli, spinach, and sea vegetables, and add sesame seeds, walnuts, Brazil nuts, flaxseed oil, low-fat yogurt, and soybeans to smoothies. Make smoothies with vitamin D–fortified, low-fat milk, rice milk, or soymilk.

If you're looking for go-to drinks to power your daily living and activity, you can't go wrong with the following:

- ✔ Peaches and Dreams (Chapter 12)
- ✔ Perfect in Pink (Chapter 12)
- ✔ Citrus and Mango Tango (Chapter 12)
- ✔ Get Up and Go (Chapter 16)
- ✔ Tropical Pick-Me-Up (Chapter 16)

Revving Up Your Sexy Vitality

You've got it, baby! If you have it, you likely have a healthy hormonal balance, because for both men and women, too little testosterone, which declines by an average of 10 percent per decade, lessens sexual vitality. The predominantly female hormones — progesterone and estrogen — also affect sexual desire in women, so deficiencies result in lower libido.

Although hormones are essential, you also need to be healthy to enjoy a sustained interest in sex. Insomnia, poor diet, drugs, alcohol, low-grade infections and ill health, and psychological issues all negatively impact your sexual drive. These sections take a closer look at how juices and smoothies can affect your hormones.

Balancing hormones

Like enzymes, hormones are chemical compounds that are produced by specific organs in your body such as the pancreas or the adrenal glands. Unlike enzymes, hormones are released directly into the blood stream. The difference between enzymes and hormones is that hormones carry specific messages to cells, and enzymes act as catalysts, assisting in the chemical reactions of the cells.

Some herbs have been used to increase overall sexual vitality. For example, chaste tree berries balance the pituitary gland and increase sexual energy when it's low.

For testosterone, zinc is important because it assists in producing both the hormone and sperm. The best juice and smoothie ingredients for getting plenty of zinc are sesame and pumpkin seeds, parsley, oats, yogurt, turnip, ginger, garlic, carrots, grapes, and cabbage. Eat scallops, turkey, and shrimp, as well as raw, cooked, or canned oysters once a week — you can even include canned oysters in smoothies.

To increase progesterone in women, wild yam has shown to be effective. You can add dried wild yam (found in natural food stores) to juice and smoothies.

Seeking out sexy nutrients

Some foods thought to be aphrodisiacs (such as oysters) hold up under scientific scrutiny and others don't. If you're eating a whole-foods diet that includes juices and smoothies, you aren't overly stressed, and you aren't taking prescription or recreational drugs, you should be pretty virile.

Probably the single most important thing you can do for your sex drive is to consume ten fruits and vegetables a day in as wide a variety as possible. This will provide essential nutrients that will balance all sorts of conditions, as well as your hormones.

Take for example, Vitamin C. It has been shown to improve sperm count, sperm motility, and sperm viability in men. It's also recommended for both men and women who want to increase sexual function. If you're eating a wide variety of fruits and vegetables, you'll be getting enough vitamin C for all your body's needs. Juicing peppers, kale, strawberries, citrus fruits, tomatoes, cabbage, and spinach will provide vitamin C.

Boosting Your Immune System

Your body is a miracle at work. It has several systems that keep it functioning, and when those systems are working at optimum capacity, so are you. One of those intricate biological networks is the immune system. This is your first line of defense against bacteria, microbes, viruses, toxins, and parasites. It consists of organs (thymus, spleen, tonsils, adenoids, lymph nodes), lymphatic vessels, and white blood cells. See Chapter 21 for a list of immune-building foods to juice or add to smoothies.

A very long list of damaging compounds — including cigarette smoke, pollution, soil and air-borne chemicals, free radicals, yeast, bacteria, fungi, parasites, stress, poor diet and nutrient deficiencies, and drugs (especially antibiotics) — all contribute to compromising your immunity.

Flushing and fueling your immune organs

In order to be and stay healthy, strengthening and maintaining a strong immune system is essential. With a weak or dysfunctional immune system, infections can invade and flourish in your body, and other illness and disease, (including cancer cells and autoimmune diseases like rheumatoid arthritis and multiple sclerosis) can develop undetected. If you're easily susceptible to colds, viruses, flu, infections, and other illnesses, this is a sign that your immunity is low.

Flushing

Taking a juice fast two to four times a year will not only flush and cleanse the digestive system, but also allow other systems, including the lymph and other immune organs, to be cleansed and brought back to optimum functioning. Juice cleansing boosts the immune response by helping to keep the immune system from overreacting and developing autoimmune responses and by speeding up the ability of the white blood cells to destroy diseased, damaged, and dead cells. See Chapter 9 for more details on cleansing and detoxifying.

Fueling

Regardless of whether you've cleansed, starting now, you'll want to stop eating high-fat, empty-calorie foods and start eating a whole-foods, balanced diet. Juicing offers the key to feeding your immune system because it provides pure nutrients in an absorbable form without stressing the digestive system. Here's how to fuel your immune system:

✔ Eat a high-fiber, low-fat diet with rich sources of low-fat proteins and omega-3 fatty acids like those found in wild salmon, flaxseed oil, walnuts, and leafy green vegetables.

✔ Eat organic foods whenever possible.

✔ Get optimum levels of vitamin D from fortified milk and milk alternative products, eggs, and shellfish, as well as from sunlight.

✔ Eat a wide assortment of at least ten fruits and vegetables every day; make sure that one-quarter to one-half of them are raw.

✔ Juice at least twice a day.

✔ Include wheatgrass, garlic, ginger, and cabbage in your daily juice.

Avoiding immune depressants

The foods you eat either support your immune system and your body or damage it. Because the gastrointestinal tract keeps out damaging molecules and pathogenic organisms, like harmful bacteria, toxins, and viruses, it's essential to support this important barrier with the foods you eat (or don't eat).

Here's a list of some substances to avoid or eliminate if you want to build a strong gastrointestinal tract and immune system:

✔ Anti-inflammatory drugs such as aspirin and ibuprofen (because constant use irritates the gastrointestinal tract)

✔ Alcohol (because it irritates the stomach lining)

✔ Red meat and fried foods (because saturated fat increases inflammation, an autoimmune response in your body that causes all sorts of problems including rheumatoid arthritis)

✔ Processed and highly refined foods with added preservatives (because they tax the immune system by negatively affecting the gastrointestinal lining without adding essential nutrients)

✔ Non-organic foods grown with pesticides (because they may damage the gastrointestinal lining)

✔ The chemicals in cigarettes (because they add toxic metals such as cadmium, lead, and mercury to the body, which severely compromises your immune system)

✔ White sugar (because it may reduce your white blood cells' ability to destroy germs)

Improving Your Memory

Everyone needs to be able to recall facts, events, and people. You want to enjoy peak mental performance (including focusing mentally and utilizing your mental capacities virtually on demand). Here again, adequate nutrition is the very first step to improving not only your memory, but also your other brain functions.

Free radical damage accounts for a large part of the general decline in mental performance, as well as causing actual brain cell damage and shrinkage of the brain itself. As proteins in the brain are attacked by free radicals, they're transformed into *lipofuscin,* a brown slime that coats the neurons. As the slime thickens, memory and other mental functions decline.

The good news is twofold:

- ✔ Flushing clears sludge in the brain, and fueling with antioxidants and other phytonutrients stops free radical damage and feeds the cells brain-building and brain-protecting compounds.

- ✔ With mental exercise, the neurological pathways in the brain can be reopened and rebuilt so that memory and other functions are restored.

All this results in improved mental performance, the ability to learn, increased recall and memory, and clear thinking, with the result that your train of thought is not impaired and your brain is working as it should.

The brain uses 20 percent of the body's energy through carbohydrates. When the brain receives a steady supply of glucose from carbohydrates in fruits and vegetables for fuel, it operates smoothly and consistently. Mental confusion, dizziness, and, in extreme cases, convulsions and lack of consciousness occur when energy is not supplied in a steady stream. Foods with a low glycemic index (see Chapter 9) keep the blood sugar levels from peaking and crashing.

Protein (especially tryptophan and tyrosine) is used to build neurotransmitters, which affect attention and learning capabilities in the brain. Fats are the major components of the brain cell membrane, so a diet rich in amino acids and omega-3 fatty acids is vital to a buff brain. Minerals are also important for brain function. For example, magnesium and manganese are both needed for brain energy; zinc is essential for protecting against aging of the brain; sodium, potassium, and calcium facilitate the transmission of messages; and iron carries oxygen to the brain cells and aids in the formation of brain neurotransmitters.

A whole-foods diet that includes plenty of raw fruits and vegetables, nuts, seeds, whole grains, legumes, lentils, and other foods like eggs, avocados, flaxseed oil, wild cold-water fatty fish, berries, and pomegranates protects the brain.

Feeding the brain

The ability to focus and concentrate is important to everyone, especially as you age. This is because, over time, effects of the environment, poor diet, and lack of exercise exact a toll on the brain and the rest of the body. Like all body organs and systems, the brain performs a myriad of functions and requires energy from carbohydrates like those found in fruits and vegetables. It also requires protein and omega-3 fatty acids for the formation of its cell structure.

In addition to specific foods for the brain, don't underestimate the power of sleep to reboot your brain. Avoid sugar because it depresses the immune function; alcohol because it suppresses your nervous system and makes you groggy; energy drinks that make you anxious and irritate the nerves; and soda because it has been shown to make people depressed and anxious.

Here's a list of some nutrients to include in smoothies and juices to feed the brain:

- **Antioxidants:** Vitamins A, C, and E hunt and destroy free radicals in the brain and the entire body. Consuming raw fruits and vegetables is the best way to ensure that you get enough antioxidants to prevent the risk of Alzheimer's disease and to slow the progression of memory loss. Specifically, berries such as wild blueberries, strawberries, and raspberries have been found to preserve memory and cut your risk of Parkinson's and Alzheimer's diseases. (See Chapter 20 for ten antioxidant-rich fruits and vegetables.)

- **Protein:** Plant protein (from nuts, seeds, legumes, soy, whole grains, fruits, and vegetables) and small amounts of low-fat meat such as eggs, chicken, fish, and dairy products like low-fat milk and yogurt will supply more than adequate amounts of amino acids and essential protein for brain power.

- **Omega-3 fatty acids:** Adding avocado and walnuts to smoothies, and flaxseed or cod liver oil to juices or smoothies, and eating wild cold-water, fatty fish like salmon and mackerel will boost these brain-friendly and essential fatty acids in your body.

- **B-complex vitamins:** Folic acid (vitamin B9) is critical for brain development (so it's a key nutrient during pregnancy) and vitamins B6 and B12 help manufacture and release chemicals in the brain known as *neurotransmitters,* the brain's messengers. Juice dark green leafy vegetables; use yogurt, oats, and milk in smoothies; and eat sardines, salmon, fish, and seafood to get plenty of B vitamins.

For top-performing brain food, add wild blueberries, strawberries, raspberries, or pomegranate seeds to juices or smoothies; use soymilk, nuts, seeds, or puréed cooked legumes in smoothies; blend avocado and walnuts into smoothies; stir ground flaxseeds into juices or smoothies, juice dark green leafy vegetables like spinach, Swiss chard, and kale; and add yogurt and oats to smoothies.

Here are five smoothie recipes in this book that are great for the brain:

- Red Vitality (Chapter 17)
- Berry Broccoli (Chapter 17)
- Coconut Green (Chapter 17)
- Spicy Tomato Mocktail (Chapter 17)
- No-jito (Chapter 17)

Herbs for memory

Herbs enhance your diet in so many ways, so growing your own or finding a great organic source of these important ingredients will be a definite asset in helping to maintain a healthy body and brain. Here are some herbs to stir into juices and smoothies that help improve cognitive function and memory, but be sure to check with your doctor before using if you're on medication because herbs have active components that can interfere with prescription drugs:

- **Peppermint:** Clears your mind and helps you focus, boosting performance.
- **Basil essential oil:** Acts as an aromatic nerve tonic, giving you a calming energy.
- **Ginkgo biloba:** Helps to improve blood flow to the brain and other organs. Medical research has proven its effectiveness in treating the early stages of memory loss. Use it in smoothies and juices along with a juice cleanse or fast as an effective memory booster.
- **Sage oil:** Helps boost production of chemicals in the brain that are known to be depleted by Alzheimer's disease.
- **Rosemary:** Prevents mutations in DNA and stimulates memory.

Chapter 8

Juices and Smoothies throughout Your Life

In This Chapter

▶ Getting the nutrients you need at every age

▶ Knowing what you need when you're pregnant

*N*o matter how young or old you are, you can benefit from juices and smoothies because the quality of your life depends on the quality of the food that sustains it. Children get off to an excellent start with pure, organic purées and juices; teenagers fuel active bodies with nutrients and energy; and seniors maintain a healthy immune system and memory while ensuring that their muscles and bones are strong.

This chapter offers everyone the potential to live long, healthy lives. It shows how a consistent diet of fresh whole foods and pure fruit and vegetable juices, along with a wide range of smoothies and supplemental ingredients, provides essential nutrients at each stage in your growth and helps you and those you care for to grasp the vitality that is everyone's birthright.

Due to hormonal changes and the needs of the growing infant, pregnant women have their own nutritional requirements. Juices and smoothies play an important role in the health of both mother and child.

If you want to really dig into the details on nutritional requirements, check out the latest edition of *Nutrition For Dummies* by Carol Ann Rinzler (John Wiley & Sons, Inc.).

Choosing Healthy Drinks for Children

Infancy and childhood are times of rapid cell division and growth. Requirements for all nutrients are higher during this stage of life than at any other developmental phase. In fact, a baby is expected to triple its birth weight and increase its length and head size by 50 percent by the end of the first year of life. This accelerated expansion of muscles, bones, and tissue continues through childhood and puberty.

Infants require up to 18 times the number of calories that sustain adults. The best "drink" you can give an infant is breast milk — it provides energy, protein, and improved immune function. Mothers who breast-feed are giving their babies the very best start in life, and breast-feeding mothers need the best nutrients for their own bodies and the milk they're producing (see the "Pumping Up the Nutrients When You're Pregnant or Breast-Feeding" section, later in this chapter).

Requirements for fatty acids are higher in infants than in adults due to their role in the development of the central nervous system. Polyunsaturated fats and fats high in omega-3 fatty acids, such as those found in plant foods, are essential to the diets of both the breast-feeding mother and her baby. Although babies can't drink smoothies, breast-feeding mothers can supplement their omega-3 fatty acids by adding flax seeds, walnuts, tofu, and even fish oil to boost this important nutrient.

As children grow, vegetable protein, vitamins, minerals, and phytonutrients are all essential in order to meet their needs. The energy needs for children ages 1 to 3 are still very high, running around 990 calories per day. After age 3, their needs drops off so that between the ages of 6 and the time they hit puberty, kids' caloric needs are based on weight, height, and physical activity.

Children ages 1 to 3 can be given pure vegetable or fruit juices that have been diluted with an equal amount of pure water. Water can be gradually reduced in the pure juice drinks for children ages 4 and older. After age 4, you can start to introduce high-energy smoothie drinks with vegetable protein from nuts, seeds, bran, avocadoes, wheat germ, and whey protein.

Start giving your kids juices and smoothies now, and you'll establish habits that will last them a lifetime.

Tackling the Needs of Teenagers

For teenagers, protein and energy are essential, but everything from vitamins A and C for skin and calcium and phosphorous for bone growth is important to maintaining an equilibrium as hormones and outside stresses take their toll.

With junk food and soft drinks so much a part of teens' life, they don't always care that pizza and soda don't make for a balanced diet. And yet, it's at this stage in their lives that teens can benefit most from establishing lasting healthy food habits that include juices and smoothies. Pure vegetable juice is perhaps the single most important food that teens can have that will ensure that they get the nutrients they need for development. Low-fat dairy smoothies slide into the number two slot in terms of delivering protein and calcium.

When menstruation starts for females, they need more iron. In teen males, vitamins C, K, and some of the B vitamins, along with choline, magnesium, zinc, chromium, and manganese, become important. Short of taking supplements, vegetable and fruit smoothies and juices are the perfect foods for keeping teenagers healthy inside and out.

In terms of daily requirements, one or two pure vegetable or fruit juices and at least one smoothie that includes a protein and a calcium source are essential for teens.

It's never too late to get your kids started drinking juices and smoothies, so don't worry if you have teenagers today and you've never juiced or made smoothies before. Start today!

Getting the Nutrients You Need as You Age

Unless you're fit and active or, at the other end of the spectrum, suffering from loss of appetite because of surgery or some other cause, you don't need as much energy from food than you did when you were younger. But that doesn't mean you don't need nutrients. Intake of high-quality nutrients in pure juice and whole foods is essential for a wide variety of health functions, including immunity, infection and disease prevention, and strengthening of muscles and bones.

Keeping fit and participating in low-impact exercise designed to maintain bone density is absolutely essential after 50.

Vitamin D is a key nutrient for those older than 70. According to the National Institutes for Health, the daily requirement is 600 IU per day from birth through the age of 70. Over the age of 70, it jumps to 800 IU per day.

Here are some tips as you age:

- Be careful not to load up on high-calorie ingredients in smoothies unless you're undernourished or underweight. Low-fat dairy and plant sources of protein (nuts, seeds, oatmeal, tofu) and vitamin D-enriched dairy foods are excellent ingredients for smoothies as you get older. Pure vegetable juice is better than fruit juice because of the high nutrient value and lower sugar content.

- You can easily take nutritional supplements and medications in smoothies because they blend in so well and don't add an unpleasant taste to the drink.

- Boosting smoothies with protein and calcium found in milk and milk products and using other healthy ingredients makes them nutritionally equal to meals. If you don't have the appetite you used to, or if you live alone and just don't feel like cooking for yourself, a smoothie can be a great way to ensure you're still getting a healthy, nutritious meal.

Pumping Up the Nutrients When You're Pregnant or Breast-Feeding

You've created a new life with your partner, and now you're the sole source of absolutely everything your fetus or baby needs. Your diet has never been as important as it is right now, and getting the vitamins, minerals, protein, carbohydrates, good fats, and phytonutrients is your job. Pure vegetable and fruit juices can be huge assets to your diet when you're pregnant or breast-feeding, helping to boost all the essential nutrients and doing it effectively and without adding fat.

Face it: Eating for two means that you need it all: energy; protein; essential fatty acids; vitamins A, C, D, E and the B vitamins (B12 in particular); folate; choline; calcium; phosphorus; magnesium; potassium; iron; zinc; copper; chromium; selenium; iodine; manganese; and molybdenum. It's a long list and one that you need to be sure to address for the health of your baby and for you.

Your doctor will give you recommendations about healthy levels of all these nutrients. The best you can do for your baby and you is to eat a wide variety of whole organic foods and choose pure vegetable and fruit juices for snacks two or three times a day. Low-fat smoothies with protein and calcium will complement these eating habits to supply what your body is using. If you're looking to add supplements to your smoothies, try avocado, flax, nuts, seeds, wheat germ, oatmeal, tofu, or whey.

For more tips on nutrition during pregnancy, check out *Pregnancy Cooking & Nutrition For Dummies,* by Tara Gidus, MS, RD (John Wiley & Sons, Inc.).

Mothers who are breast-feeding, perhaps more than any other group of people, may benefit the most from smoothies and juices. This is because new mothers need to replenish stores of minerals (like iron and calcium) in their own bodies and they require protein, as well as essential vitamins and phytonutrients, in order to produce high-energy, high-nutrient milk for their babies. Drinking pure fruit and vegetable juices two or three times a day is ideal.

Deciding Whether Smoothies and/or Juices Are Right for You

If you're making your health a top priority now, you're not alone. Trends toward healthier options in all areas of our lives are peaking, with the biggest population bulge, the Baby Boomers, reaching 50 or older. And these trends are filtering down to younger generations as well, so that juicing and smoothies have become a significant part of a healthy daily diet.

According to the American Heart Association (AHA), heart disease is the number-one killer of Americans. The AHA says that you can reduce your risk of heart disease by the foods you eat and drink; it identifies seven health and lifestyle factors that impact health and quality of life. If you visit the AHA website (www.heart.org), you can start getting healthy by checking out My Life Check. In the meantime, here are the AHA's seven health factors:

- ✔ Don't smoke.
- ✔ Maintain a healthy weight for your sex and age.
- ✔ Engage in regular physical activity.
- ✔ Eat natural, whole foods and avoid high-fat, high-sugar, fast- and refined-foods.

✔ Manage your blood pressure, preferably by diet and exercise.

✔ Watch and manage cholesterol.

✔ Keep blood sugar, or glucose, at healthy levels.

In one way or another, juices and smoothies can help with many of these factors. One place to start to determine if juices or smoothies are a viable lifestyle option for you is to take the personal health questionnaire in the nearby sidebar. You can use it to gauge whether you're getting the appropriate amounts of fruits and vegetables.

Taking stock: A personal health questionnaire

Setting your own personal health goals is an excellent way to put a focus on diet, physical activity, and mental attitude. A good place to start with your diet is to honestly answer the questions in this section and measure your answers against the facts from health experts. This points out any discrepancy between what's ideal and where you are right now, and it can help you to take the steps you need to have a healthy life.

1. **How do you take your meals?**

   a. **Do you eat breakfast?** Eating breakfast is essential to supplying nutrients to the cells for the workday ahead.

   b. **If so, what do you eat for breakfast?** Fresh fruits or vegetables, small amount of protein, and some source of omega-3 acids are best to start the day.

2. **What beverages do you drink in a day?** Coffee, regular tea, and soft drinks don't contribute to a healthy diet. Eight glasses of water is optimal.

3. **What snacks do you eat between meals and when do you eat them?** Keeping a log of exactly what you eat for a whole week will point out what kinds of foods you go to when you feel down or bored or hungry.

4. **How often do you go through the drive-through in a week?** It should be a rare to never occurrence.

5. **How often do you eat fast food (burgers, tacos, deep-fried chicken, pizza, french fries)?** It should be a rare-to-never occurrence.

6. **How many home-cooked dinners do you eat in a week?** It should be a five- to seven-days-a-week occurrence.

7. **How many fruits and vegetables do you eat in a day?** Studies show that eating seven and ideally ten or more servings of fruits and vegetables (with vegetables being five or more of those servings) lowers the risk of many modern diseases.

If your diet is falling short of a healthy, preventive, whole foods way of eating, changes are in order.

Remember: Substituting fresh fruit or vegetable juices or smoothies for high-calorie, high-fat snacks and drinks is one of the easiest ways to improve your diet. If you're already having fresh fruit for snacks, great! Try fresh vegetable drinks, and expand your choices. Only you can determine what, when, and how you'll eat and drink.

Chapter 9

Preventing Diseases with Juices and Smoothies

I *can improve my health and lower my risk of modern diseases through diet.* I believe that statement to be absolutely true. And health experts from all areas of study and practice are backing the concept up with solid science. Doctors T. Colin Campbell and Caldwell Esselstyn (advocates of a low-fat, whole-food, plant-based diet or Forks over Knives for combating cancers, diabetes, and heart disease) have spent their professional careers debunking the common myths surrounding the foods that people think they require. These myths are, namely: animal protein is essential; calcium from milk is the best way to have strong bones; carbohydrates are bad; organic, healthy foods are an expensive fad. Through human studies and observing global health statistics, and by working with heart patients, they have proved beyond a doubt that a diverse, plant-based diet high in vegetables, fruits, nuts, whole grains, legumes and herbs, one that is low or completely devoid of animal and dairy foods holds the key to being and staying in good health.

First up, protein: Plant foods contain sufficient protein for all your needs and when you consume a wide range of whole plant foods, you satisfy your body's requirement for 8 to 10 percent total daily calories from protein. That's it. That's all you need and the protein quality is better from plants because animal proteins have been linked directly to cancer, heart disease, diabetes, Alzheimer's disease and kidney stones.

Calcium from kale, broccoli, bok choy, sea vegetables, beans, and Brussels sprouts comes with a plethora of phytonutrients including vitamin K, phytates, and antioxidants, which makes it better in many ways (because it is in a useable form) than milk for strong bones and preventing osteoporosis (low bone density).

Not all carbohydrates are alike. Carbohydrates from a whole foods diet provide fiber, essential fatty acids, B vitamins, zinc and protein, while those from refined, processed foods can raise triglycerides, promote weight gain, and increase blood sugar. The difference between the two means operating at optimum healthy levels or being on the slippery slope downwards.

Incorporating more plant foods in your glass and on your plate means crowding out expensive meat and dairy products. Using pulp from juicing in soup, stew, baked goods, and smoothies adds fiber and nutrients and it means there is no waste.

Living Longer

It's a fact of life: Eventually, all living things die. No matter what you eat or drink, you can't stop or avoid your own mortality. Sounds terminal, but the good news is this: You do have some influence over when and how you'll die.

Science reports that people can actually extend both the quality and the length of their lives if they enjoy health-supporting foods in the right amounts and engage in moderate, regular exercise. I don't know about you, but for some people I've spoken to about diet and exercise, it's almost a letdown for them to discover that the key to the live-longer, look-younger, feel-better dream is as close as eating a balanced, whole-food diet and doing some form of aerobic exercise for 30 minutes every day. It's incredibly simple, but, for some reason, many people seem to want a magic pill or potion from the fabled fountain of youth.

If you could only change one thing in your diet, adding a daily, pure fruit or vegetable juice and/or smoothie would be the best possible thing you could do. This is because raw fruits and vegetables are loaded with antioxidants, those nutrients that protect cells from the damaging effects of free radicals. Free radicals, which are part of the normal body processes and are found in processed foods, chemicals, and air-borne toxins, contribute in a major way to the aging process because they weaken cells and allow illness and disease to grow.

Science has pinpointed free radical damage as a link in the debilitating diseases of aging such as atherosclerosis, diabetes, rheumatoid arthritis, Alzheimer's disease, Parkinson's disease, cataracts, and cancer. The one proven way to stop the chain reaction of free radicals attacking healthy cells and turning them into more free radicals is to unleash a steady stream of antioxidants (such as vitamins A, C and E) into the bloodstream. Providing a steady supply of pure antioxidants by drinking juices and smoothies at least twice in a day means that those nutrients are ready for absorption into the blood consistently and immediately.

Your diet, including fresh fruit smoothies and juices, and your choice to include moderate exercise daily are the two most important things you have complete control over. This is where you must start if you want to live a long and productive life.

Following some guidelines to longevity

You can skip this sidebar if you want to increase your chances of disease and dying young. On the other hand, if you want to live a long and healthy life, the ideas in the following list can help you get there:

✔ **Eat ten fresh, raw, organic fruits and vegetables every day.** Make juices and smoothies part of your daily routine because studies show that the nutrients in fruits and vegetables protect against modern diseases.

✔ **Rejuvenate your body, especially your organs of digestion, by going on a juice fast at least four times per year.** Fasting allows your liver, kidneys, and lymph system to rest and renew. (See Chapter 10 for more on fasting.)

✔ **Maintain your ideal weight by eating small portions of whole foods including fruit, vegetables, legumes, whole grains, nuts, seeds, lentils, and very small amounts of low-fat dairy products and lean meats.** Studies show that obesity shortens lifespan.

✔ **Avoid sugar, alcohol, caffeine, and nicotine.** Research indicates that high sugar levels speed the aging process. Smoking generates free radicals and causes cancer.

✔ **Cleanse your liver, colon, stomach, intestines, and kidneys.** Keeping these organs of elimination in optimum condition will lengthen your lifespan. See Chapter 10 for a cleansing plan or juice fast that will help colon, stomach, intestines, and kidneys.

Keeping Your Blood Sugar Under Control to Prevent and Manage Diabetes

Diabetes is a lifelong, chronic disease that is caused by too little insulin or a resistance to insulin. Insulin is a hormone produced by the pancreas to move blood sugar (called *glucose*) from the bloodstream into muscle, fat, and liver cells where it can be used as fuel.

There are two main types of diabetes (type 1 and type 2), as well as a condition called *gestational diabetes,* which is high blood sugar during pregnancy in a woman who doesn't have diabetes.

Because diabetes affects so many people (more than 20 million Americans), and because type 2 diabetes most often occurs in adulthood and is linked to diet and obesity, nutritionists are concentrating their efforts on diet and exercise to reduce the risk of this deadly disease, for which there is no cure.

There is no way to prevent type 1 diabetes. Maintaining an ideal body weight, healthy diet, and an active lifestyle may prevent type 2 diabetes and will help manage type 1 diabetes.

There is no set diet for diabetics, but keeping blood glucose levels on target by making wise food choices and staying physically active is the best plan. Smoothies and juices can be an important part of a healthy, whole-food diet. Because they're so much higher in natural sugars, fruit juices and

The glycemic index and you

The glycemic index (GI) is a ranking of foods on a scale from 0 to 100. The number assigned to each food is an indication of how much they raise a person's blood sugar level. Foods that have a high GI raise blood sugar the most; foods with a low GI raise blood sugar the least. The goal, particularly for people with diabetes, is to stick to low-GI foods (those with a GI of about 55 or less).

Juicing, by its very nature, eliminates the fiber from fruits and vegetables, which means that

juices have a higher GI than the whole fruits or vegetables do. If you have diabetes, you should drink fresh fruit juice only in small amounts and stick to juicing low-GI vegetables.

For much more information on the glycemic index, check out *The Glycemic Index Diet For Dummies,* by Meri Raffetto, RD, LDN (John Wiley & Sons, Inc.).

smoothies are *not* the best choice for diabetics. In addition, you need to be aware of glycemic levels of some vegetables when you're planning to make vegetable juices or smoothies (see the nearby sidebar for more on the glycemic index).

Smoothies that are made with liquids other than juice, that are low in calories, and that have some low-fat protein make excellent snack choices for people with diabetes.

Getting a Hold on Heart Health

The way to a healthy heart is through your stomach. And what goes into your stomach starts out on your plate or in your glass. So it makes sense to pay attention to the crucial elements–vitamins, minerals, fiber and phytonutri- ents–in food that help prevent cardiovascular disease. Of course, where do these heart healthy nutrients come from? You betcha: plants. Are you seeing a pattern here? Again and again, the path to a healthy body follows a whole food diet, one that is rich in vegetables, fruit, nuts, seeds, legumes, whole grains, and herbs.

Eating a predominantly plant-based diet is one of the most important things you can do to reduce your risk of heart disease and the other major modern diseases. Here's how a healthy diet will foster heart and general overall health:

✔ Increasing the nutrients your body needs from fruit, vegetables, legumes, whole grains, herbs, nuts, and seeds

✔ Managing your weight because plant foods are lower in calories

✔ Keeping your blood pressure at a healthy level

✔ Controlling blood sugar levels and cholesterol with fiber

✔ Boosting your overall feeling of wellness, energy and vitality

✔ Making you look good and feel better about yourself

Lowering your cholesterol with pulp

As you know by now, dietary fiber is found exclusively in plant foods — fruits, vegetables, whole grains, and legumes. Eating fiber is one of the easiest and least expensive ways to lower cholesterol, prevent disease, and maintain health because it helps the body to eliminate waste materials and deadly toxins. Water-soluble fiber lowers cholesterol and stabilizes blood sugar.

This is all great news, but don't juices and smoothies remove all that fiber? Yes and no. The fiber in fruits and vegetables is removed during juicing when the pulp is separated from the juice. But you can freeze that pulp and add it to soups, stews, and baked goods like muffins, and you can blend it into smoothies. (For more ways to use pulp, see Chapter 14.) Even though they're liquidized or finely chopped in smoothies, whole fruits and vegetables contain both water-soluble and insoluble fiber from those plants. The fiber is simply liquidized so that you can drink the ingredients, but it's still there; in fact, blending hard fruits and vegetables actually saves your digestive system that job.

Bottom line: The National Cholesterol Education Program says that along with a whole-foods diet and regular exercise, 10 to 25 grams of soluble fiber a day will lower cholesterol.

Here's how to increase soluble fiber in your diet:

- Drink juice for concentrated boosts of nutrients, but save the pulp and use it in cooking or add it to smoothies.
- Drink raw fruit and vegetable smoothies.
- Stir psyllium into juices, and add nuts, seeds, cooked beans, bran, and oats to smoothies.
- Eat raw, high-fiber fruits and vegetables — apples, oranges, berries, pears, figs, prunes, broccoli, cauliflower, Brussels sprouts, and carrots.
- Include whole grains, legumes, and lentils on a regular basis.

Here are five fiber boosters to get you going:

- Banana Breakfast (Chapter 16)
- Berry Nutty (Chapter 16)
- Green Energy Breakfast (Chapter 17)
- Vita-E (Chapter 17)
- Peas and Carrots (Chapter 17)

Limiting unhealthy fats

Saturated and trans fats are a contributing factor to coronary artery disease because they raise blood cholesterol. High blood cholesterol can lead to atherosclerosis (a buildup of plaques in your arteries), which clogs the insides of the arteries, causing blockages to the flow of blood and ultimately increasing your risk of heart attack and stroke.

The best way to reduce saturated and trans fats is to eat less animal protein and increase the fruit and vegetables you consume. Avoid solid fats–butter, margarine, shortening, and animal fats in meat and dairy–and cook with mono-unsaturated fats such as extra-virgin olive oil or a medium-chain fatty acid such as coconut oil.

Preventing and Managing Cancers

Learning to recognize the foods that either discourage or encourage the growth of cancer cells is critical to your health, but it's not complicated. Basically, as I have been saying over and over in this book, eating a plant-based diet consisting of whole foods including fresh vegetables, fruit, peas, beans and legumes, whole grains, nuts and herbs will supply free radical fighting antioxidants that protect and repair tissue at the cellular level. These foods also build, repair, heal, and perform a myriad of other finely designed functions that are all aimed at supporting your immune system and preventing diseases, including cancer.

Specifically, here are the nutrients and foods that discourage the growth and proliferation of cancer:

✔ **Plant proteins:** Getting your daily requirement of protein from plants is not difficult when you follow a whole foods diet. Avoiding animal protein from meats (especially red meats such as beef, pork and lamb), eggs and dairy foods is critical to preventing and lowering detected cancers.

Juice a wide variety of fresh vegetables and fruits, and eat or blend whole grains, legumes, nuts, and seeds in vegetable and fruit smoothies to get plenty of protein along with calcium, vitamins and other phytonutrients.

✔ **Antioxidants:** Today's stressful life combined with the natural process of metabolizing food to energy releases free radicals, which can damage cells. Antioxidants neutralize deadly free radicals.

To get plenty of antioxidants, juice and blend brightly colored fruit and vegetables, and eat whole grains and nuts or add them to smoothies.

✔ **Anthocyanins:** Super nutrients that are antioxidant and anti-inflammatory, two of the most important factors in preventing diseases such as cancer, Alzheimer's, Parkinson's, diabetes, aging, arthritis and heart disease. Dark red, purple or blue fruit and vegetables are highest in anthocyanins but brightly colored fruits and vegetables offer excellent quantities.

Juice and blend a variety of berries, red and green vegetables and add anti-inflammatory herbs such as ginger, turmeric, cinnamon, garlic, chamomile, basil, and cayenne.

✔ **Fiber:** The parts of plants that your body can't digest are important in keeping your digestive system clean and healthy by pushing out waste and toxins before they can turn carcinogenic.

To bulk up on fiber, eat whole, raw vegetables and fruit, whole grains, nuts, beans, peas and legumes, and drink smoothies made with those ingredients.

Other cancer risk-reduction factors include the following:

✔ **Avoiding sugars:** Cancer cells feed on sugar, using vast amounts of glucose for energy and as building blocks for cell replication. When you eat a processed food, high-fat diet laced with refined white sugars and flours and heaps of chemicals, you're feeding cancer cells if they exist in your body. And even if cancer isn't present in your cells, you're exposing both them and your tissues to the threat from free radicals.

Low-glycemic vegetable juices and smoothies flush your cells with pure, absorbable nutrients, releasing free radical fighting antioxidants without natural sugars.

✔ **Avoiding smoking and alcohol:** Smoking can lead to cancer. Alcohol feeds sugars directly into the blood and lowers your will to make wise diet choices.

✔ **Lowering stress:** Stress constantly drains the body's ability to renew, replace, and refresh itself, opening up a lowered defense system for cancer cells to develop.

✔ **Watching your meat intake:** Keep meat to a minimum and eat only small amounts of chicken or fish (the portion should be able to fit in the palm of your hand) occasionally — about two or three times a week.

✔ **Making wise choices about oils.** Choose polyunsaturated fats like extra-virgin olive oil or medium-chain fatty acids, such as coconut oil. Avoid any foods with hydrogenated or partially hydrogenated oils.

✔ **Eating more fruits and veggies:** Consume at least five and preferably 10 vegetables and fruits every day.

Chapter 10

Juicing to Cleanse or Detoxify

Environmental toxins are everywhere: in the water, soil, air, and food. Even the normal metabolic functions that go on inside your body create waste and some level of toxins. Eating organic food and avoiding processed and refined foods helps, but for anyone living in this fast-paced, stress-filled, modern society, regular juice cleansing and detoxifying have become a necessary part of a healthy lifestyle.

In this chapter, I explain the difference between cleansing and detoxifying and offer guidelines for doing both.

Cleansing: Clearing Waste from Your Digestive System

Cleansing is all about removing waste from your digestive system, as well as your organs and other tissues. For this process, you use specific fruits, vegetables, and/or herbs to stimulate the body to eliminate stored waste and toxins. Cleansing usually is done with herbal teas and fresh fruit juices and doesn't necessarily involve *fasting* (complete abstinence from food).

In the strictest sense of the term, *fasting* is abstaining from all food while drinking only water. Fasting with only water is a severe step and should be undertaken only with the help and consent of your health practitioner.

You don't need to abstain from food while cleansing. However, eating only raw fruits and vegetables (in salads) is the best support you can give your body if you really want to cleanse at the cellular level. Eating a high-fat, low-fiber diet is one of the reasons for cleansing in the first place, so it wouldn't make sense to consume anything other than organic whole foods while cleansing.

An alternative to the strict fasting is *juice fasting,* in which you abstain from food but drink raw fruit and/or vegetable juices, as well as water, for short periods of time. Technically, you aren't actually fasting if you're drinking juice, but because you're absorbing nutrients directly into the bloodstream and feeding and reconstituting the cells without actually using the digestive system, juice fasting is considered a form of fasting.

Considering the cleansing power of fruits

Using fruit juice to cleanse assists your body in the work it already does to eliminate toxic substances. The accumulation of stress, chemicals, and refined foods can overwhelm the organs of the digestive system (which is the system most closely connected to clearing waste). When the digestive system is overtaxed, waste accumulates and is stored in the liver, kidneys, colon, gallbladder, fat cells, bones, and other tissues. Stored toxins in your body lead to everything from sluggishness to disease (if they're allowed to build up).

The cleansing acids found in fruits

Fruits are well-known tools for cleansing and deep-cell flushing. Fruits work as cleansers because of the fiber and acids they contain. Among the acids found in fruit, three are most prevalent; in fact, they give fruit their distinct tang:

✔ **Malic acid:** Perhaps the most important cleansing acid, malic acid is an important cleanser because it's antiseptic, protecting the intestines, kidneys, liver, and stomach. It also increases energy level, protects muscles from fatigue, increases muscle performance, promotes nerve functioning, improves mental clarity, and decreases the toxic effects of aluminum and lead. Apples are a rich source of malic acid, but malic acid also is found in apricots, bananas,

cherries, grapes, lemons, peaches, plums, and prunes.

✔ **Citric acid:** My mouth starts to pucker when I think of the sour-tasting citric acid found in lemons, limes, grapefruit, oranges, pineapples, and other fruits. Food chemists use citric acid as a natural flavoring and preservative. When you consume foods with citric acid, it's absorbed into the bloodstream and excreted in your urine.

✔ **Tartaric acid:** Tartaric acid acts as an antioxidant and laxative and plays an important part in the cleansing and detoxifying process. Tartaric acid is found in grapes, tamarinds, and bananas.

Here are some fruits used for cleansing:

- ✔ **Apples:** Malic acid draws out heavy metals, such as lead and aluminum. Pectin forms a gel that absorbs and dissolves toxins and stimulates elimination. ***Note:*** Use only organic, unsprayed, unwaxed apples. If you can't find organic apples, be sure to peel them.

- ✔ **Cherries:** Cherries reduce the acidity of the blood, which makes them effective for gout and arthritis. You can mix cherry juice with equal parts apple juice or pure water.

- ✔ **Cranberries:** Cranberries are a natural diuretic and bladder and urinary tract cleanser. Mix one part cranberry juice with three parts apple juice or pure water.

- ✔ **Grapes:** Grapes are rich in tartaric acid, an antioxidant and laxative. They stimulate metabolism, which helps burn excess food and waste. They also stimulate the liver to increase its cleansing activity. ***Note:*** Use only organic red and green grapes and seeds for juice. Mix grape juice with lemon juice to reduce the sweetness.

- ✔ **Lemons:** Lemons are high in vitamin C and citric acid, making them a strong cleanser. Drink the juice of half a lemon in 8 ounces of pure water every day upon rising, before breakfast, to cleanse the stomach and small intestine. ***Note:*** Leave the white pith on for juicing. You can include one-quarter to one-half lemon with other fruit in cleansing juices.

- ✔ **Papayas:** Papayas contain papain, which digests protein, thus helping prepare the stomach and intestines for cleansing. Papayas are a laxative and clean the kidneys, liver, and intestines.

- ✔ **Pineapples:** Pineapples are high in *bromelain,* which breaks down proteins, thus aiding digestion.

- ✔ **Watermelons:** Watermelons are high in pure water and are used as a kidney and bladder cleanser. Use the red and white flesh, seeds, and rind for juice.

Cleansing without fasting

You can choose to perform a general cleanse or one that targets specific organs or systems of the body, and you can do it in a very gentle way that's non-intrusive. Simply drink a fruit juice for breakfast and again midmorning; using some of the fruits in the preceding section will start to have the desired effect (while eating a whole-foods diet the rest of the day). You can do this for several days or for two to three weeks.

If you add some of the following herbs, and combine the breakfast and mid-morning juices with a raw vegetable lunch, a midafternoon vegetable juice or smoothie, and a light vegetarian dinner, the cleanse will be even more effective:

- **Alfalfa:** Purifies the blood; nourishes the cells.
- **Burdock root:** Supports the liver, lymph glands, and digestive system; facilitates cleansing by stimulating urine and sweat.
- **Corn silk:** A diuretic that helps to flush the kidneys.
- **Dandelion leaves:** Support the liver, gallbladder, and kidney.
- **Dandelion root:** Cleanses the liver and blood; stimulates bile secretion; works as a laxative.
- **Licorice root:** A laxative that aids in elimination of waste.
- **Milk thistle:** Helps strengthen liver cells and bile secretion.
- **Red clover:** Purifies the blood; nourishes the cells.

Eat only organic whole foods and try to make at least one meal raw while you're cleansing. Don't eat sugar, dairy, refined foods, meats, or saturated fats during a cleanse or on the day immediately before or the day immediately after cleansing.

Cleansing with a juice fast

Brief periods of drinking only fresh fruit and/or vegetable juices and plenty of pure water can be a healthy way to give your digestive system a complete rest so that your body can do the toxin elimination and organ repair work it's designed to do. Juice fasts are healthy because

- Your cells are being nourished, not starved.
- Your organs of elimination aren't working to digest food, so they can focus on clearing out built-up debris and start to move toxins stored deep in fat and other tissues.

Noting the benefits of a juice fast

Finding the discipline and determination within yourself to exert self-control and forgo solid food in order to fast on fresh raw juices for at least one full day is exhilarating in itself. It spurs confidence that you can have greater control over your lifestyle decisions and diet. The effect of being cleansed or feeling flushed actually makes me want to continue eating lightly and taking juices long after the juice fast is officially over. The long-term effect is that it keeps me committed to choosing a green lifestyle; eating only organic foods; and eating whole fruits, vegetables, legumes, nuts, seeds, whole grains, chicken, and fish (while being careful about the kind and amount of dairy and meat I consume).

Immediately after a juice fast, I always experience a physical and mental high — the *juice high*. Some people shed pounds while juice fasting. I tend to shrink around the middle, the puffiness in my eyelids and ankles disappears, the stiffness in my knees goes away, I enjoy a lot more energy, the skin on my face tightens and clears, and the dark circles under my eyes are noticeably lightened. I wake up bright, alert, and with more calm readiness for all sorts of tasks that I usually put off. It feels as if a low-grade kind of depression has lifted and I'm content and happy with my life and myself.

Knowing how often to do a juice fast

Many people choose to fast using only fresh, raw juice one day every week. Others choose to use juice fasts when preparing to focus on a mental task (for example, before studying for an important test). Most people use the changing seasons or other significant markers (a birthday or other anniversary) to take a personal time-out and use a juice fast to bring the mental, spiritual, and physical aspects of their being into balance. Some people I know actually go on a retreat and combine meditation with other forms of reflection. All these ways of juice fasting are excellent preventive measures for ensuring overall health, physical energy, and mental clarity.

I enjoy a two- or three-day juice fast every year at around the summer and winter solstices.

Understanding how long to fast

As with any new change, it's always best to start slowly and build up to longer periods of juice fasting. If you're new to juicing, allow at least a month of experimenting with the recipes in this book, trimming your diet to a whole-foods approach, and finding your own level of tolerance for the pure, raw enzymes and phytonutrients your body will be getting before you even consider a juice fast. If you've spent years indulging in a high-fat, low-fiber diet with or without alcohol, drugs, and other chemical exposure, you're going to feel the punch of this new way of living.

After you're used to juicing, start your first juice fast with one or two days at the most. When you see what's involved and how you feel afterward, you can decide how often and when you want to enjoy your juice fast regimen. Stick with one or two days every year or every few months if you like. Or start to increase the time by one day each fast. You shouldn't do a juice fast for more than five days unless you're working with a health practitioner.

Deciding who should decline from fasting

If you're pregnant or breast-feeding, a juice fast isn't advised. People who are recovering from illness or surgery should check with their healthcare provider before juice fasting. Growing children or teenagers who are eating a whole food, fruit, and vegetable-rich diet don't benefit from juice fasting. However, obese teens or those suffering from acne may find juice fasting to be beneficial for the reasons I outline in this chapter.

Teens and young adults may need supervision with juice fasting in order to prevent unhealthy habits from developing and to guard against diet extremes that may lead to anorexia.

Juice fasting, step by step

In order for a juice fast to be effective, you need to do it right. In this section, I walk you through each phase of a juice fast, starting in the weeks leading up to it.

A few weeks before the juice fast

I start a few weeks in advance by mentally preparing for a juice fast. I like to have personal downtime while juice fasting, so I usually choose to do it over a long weekend. I mark the date on my calendar and keep the actual juice fast days clear of any obligations. When I've selected and blocked off the actual days for juice fasting, I focus some mental energy on visualizing what I'll be doing to fill the days and evenings and what functions the fruits, vegetables, and herbs will be accomplishing in my body.

The week before the juice fast

The week before, I may clean my house, organize my music, or get in some books I've wanted to read. I tell my family and friends that this is my "cleanse weekend" so they know I won't want to have dinner at a restaurant or go to a party.

It's not that you can't do anything while fasting. I just choose to do reflective things that bring me inner peace when I fast. I often conduct a juice fast with my husband. One summer, I enjoyed the process with a close friend at her cottage.

Two days before the juice fast

Prepare a list of whole foods, fruits, vegetables, and herbs that you'll be consuming before, during, and after the juice fast. Shop for, clean, and store them so they're ready when you need to prepare the light, raw meals and use them in the actual juice fast.

The day before the juice fast

Eat only raw foods and don't eat any dairy or meat products. You can prepare a smoothie for breakfast and a fruit or vegetable salad using a dressing of one part raw nut or avocado oil to two parts lemon or lime juice for lunch and dinner. Snack on raw fruits or vegetables and raw, unsalted nuts and seeds. If you have a high-performance blender, you can prepare a hot soup using vegetables.

For recipes for raw meals, check out *Raw Food For Dummies,* by Cherie Soria and Dan Ladermann (John Wiley & Sons, Inc.), and *Clean Up Your Diet,* by Max Tomlinson (Sterling Publishing).

During the fast

You're mentally ready and you have all the ingredients for your day or two of juice fasting. Now it's easy: Simply make yourself a fresh juice four to six times every day. You can choose to have only fruit or only vegetable juices, or you may decide to have pure fruit juices until noon and then vegetable (or a combination of fruit and vegetable) juices after noon. The important thing is that you don't eat anything during the days of the fast.

Drink eight glasses of pure water or water with pure lemon juice added and, if you like, herbal teas. Light exercise such as walking, stretching, dancing, gardening, or yoga is great during juice fasting. You can go to work if you need to and you can socialize — just don't do strenuous exercise/work or put yourself in a stressful situation.

To facilitate toxin release, do the following:

- **Every morning of your fast, use a dry loofah sponge or a natural bristle brush to dry-brush your body all over.** Take a shower and then rinse under cool water.

- **Every morning of your fast, take a warm water enema.** Because you aren't eating solids and the fiber isn't helping eliminate food, you'll benefit from an enema, which injects the liquid into the rectum to help release food from it.

- **Be sure to drink a minimum of eight glasses of water every day.** Drinking eight glasses of water during a juice fast is critical in helping your body to dilute and eliminate toxins.

- **Each evening of your fast, take a full-soak bath.** Fill the tub with hot water that's comfortable to sit in and add 1 cup of baking soda and the juice of 3 lemons to the water. Immerse your entire body in the water for 30 to 90 minutes, topping up with hot water as the water cools.

You may experience headache and slight depression during a juice fast, especially if you're used to coffee and alcohol or junk foods loaded with chemicals. These feelings will pass, but it could take three or four days. By juice fasting and allowing your digestive organs to rest, the toxins stored in them and in other body tissues are released back into your bloodstream where they can do damage all over again. But because you aren't eating solid food, your kidneys, liver, gallbladder, and spleen can deal with the reappearing waste. Pure water is essential in helping to dilute and move these chemicals out of your body.

You also may experience minor aches or sore muscles, temporary exhaustion, loss of appetite, runny nose, acne, body odor, and bad breath. These symptoms will pass, and you'll begin to have the opposite reaction — your skin will clear and other minor irritations will disappear. If you feel more than uncomfortable during a fast, discontinue it and resume a light, whole-foods diet.

The day after the juice fast

You did it, congratulations! You feel great, like you could do this forever. Or maybe you're ravenous and feel as if you could eat a horse. Either way, go gently back to eating and promise yourself that this is the start of a healthy lifestyle.

The day after the juice fast, eat only raw foods and don't eat any dairy or meat products. You can prepare breakfast, snacks, and a fruit or vegetable salad as explained in the earlier "The day before the juice fast," section.

Detoxifying: Ridding Your Body of Toxins

While cleansing zeroes in on clearing your digestive system of toxic waste from various causes, detoxifying focuses solely on flushing toxins like heavy metals and other chemical substances from your tissues and organs.

Although cleansing is great, you may want to take it one step further to actually detoxify your body. Although the terms *cleansing* and *detoxifying* are often used interchangeably, detoxing is a program that targets specific toxins and areas of the body and is usually longer and more intense than cleansing.

The body processes toxins through the kidneys and liver, and excretes them through the urine, feces, breath, and sweat. When those organs and flushing mechanisms become clogged, the body begins to store dangerous toxic substances in the kidneys, liver, fat, and even bone cells, among other places. Although it's always best to avoid breathing, drinking, or eating toxic chemicals, you can't always do this, so that's where a thorough detoxifying program comes in.

Detoxing is always helpful, but there's not much point in doing it if you're only going to return to a lifestyle full of toxic substances (both in the foods you eat and in the environment you live in). If you're not serious about making changes to your diet and your home, you should probably skip the rest of this chapter.

Identifying toxic substances

High amounts of polychlorinated biphenyls (PCBs), herbicides, and pesticides (such as DDT) have been found in the livers of people who are exposed to them. Your kidneys are susceptible to toxins as well, which can cause weakness, sluggishness, and poor performance. When these organs slow down, and especially if the colon becomes congested, toxins will be stored or (in the case of an ill-functioning colon) leak back into the bloodstream. When one or all of these digestive organs are compromised, nutrients are not absorbed and your entire body suffers, with malnutrition a real threat.

So, how can you tell if you have high levels of toxic substances in your body? You should have a pretty good idea if you smoke or take drugs or eat a poor diet. And the symptoms listed in the following section will help you to pinpoint some of the symptoms of toxicity.

But if you still want scientific proof, several laboratory tests are useful in detecting toxins in the body. For example, hair mineral analysis measures chronic exposure to heavy metals, while blood and fatty tissue samples may be tested to measure toxic chemical exposure found in food. If you're concerned and want to have some concrete indication of the buildup of these damaging elements, consult your healthcare provider to determine the best way to proceed.

Table 10-1 lists some of the most prevalent toxic substances that are present in our bodies in varying quantities depending on your work, diet, lifestyle, and environment.

Understanding why you should deal with toxins in the body

Everybody is exposed to chemicals through pesticides, antibiotics and hormones in food, chemicals from food packaging, household cleaners and detergents, food additives, heavy metals, pollution, drugs, cigarette smoke, recycled air (through air conditioning that reroutes chemicals from building materials), and a host of personal care products (including perfumes, soaps, and shampoo).

Table 10-1	Effects of Toxic Substances on the Body	
Toxin	**Where It's Stored**	**What It Does**
Heavy metals, such as lead, mercury, nickel, cadmium, arsenic, and aluminum	Brain, kidneys, and immune system	Early signs include headache, fatigue, muscle pains, indigestion, tremors, anemia, constipation, dizziness, and poor coordination. These signs increase with toxicity. Heavy metals also are associated with learning disabilities and other behavioral problems.
Chemicals such as food additives, drugs, alcohol, solvents, pesticides, and herbicides	Adipose tissue (fat cells), liver, spleen, and other body tissue	Can cause depression, headaches, mental confusion, mental illness, tingling in extremities, tics, and other abnormal nerve reflexes. Eating organic foods greatly reduces exposure.
Protein waste	Adipose tissue (fat cells), liver, spleen, and other body tissue	When protein (especially animal protein, meat, and dairy products) is metabolized, ammonia and urea are the waste byproducts. The kidneys are key to eliminating these wastes. Drinking eight glasses of water and/or pure juice and cutting meat intake will reduce this toxic buildup.
Bacteria and yeast from food and water and sometimes from bile	Gut and colon	Microbial toxins are linked to liver and thyroid problems, Crohn's disease, ulcerative colitis, psoriasis, allergies, asthma, and immune disorders.

Although any one of these things in small doses isn't horrible, it's the cumulative load, called the *body burden,* that has been collecting in your cells (if you've done nothing to stop it) that becomes dangerous with age. This accumulation of toxins is linked with hormonal imbalance, impaired immune function, nutritional deficiency, and an inefficient metabolism. Because toxins are stored in fat cells (mostly because they are stable and don't release the deadly chemicals into the bloodstream or other tissue, unless you cleanse or lose weight), the body begins to retain water as a precaution for diluting the toxins within its tissues. It follows that the more toxic you are, the more weight you gain and retain.

If you suffer from nine or more of the following conditions, a detox program may be beneficial for you:

- ✔ Lacking energy for daily tasks; feeling tired, sluggish, or lethargic
- ✔ Having difficulty concentrating on tasks or staying focused
- ✔ Easily catching colds, flu, and other viral or bacterial illnesses
- ✔ Having bad breath or body odor
- ✔ Having allergies or the tendency to get congested, stuffed up, or have post-nasal drip
- ✔ Experiencing bloating, gas, or indigestion after eating
- ✔ Having dark circles under your eyes
- ✔ Having eczema, acne, or psoriasis
- ✔ Often going for more than one day without having a bowel movement
- ✔ Usually drinking less than three cups of water every day (or drinking from plastic bottles on a regular basis)
- ✔ Usually eating meat two or more times a day
- ✔ Eating refined, processed foods and less than one serving of vegetables a day
- ✔ Smoking or living with a smoker
- ✔ Being exposed to industrial chemicals either by using them as solvents or cleaners, in the water or air, by swallowing them, or through accidental poisoning

If you have any of these symptoms, talk with your healthcare provider because they may be related to other serious illnesses.

If you're considering a detox program, especially if it will last more than a few days, consult your healthcare provider so that your health isn't compromised due to preexisting conditions.

Zeroing in on the best detoxifying juices

Simply moving to a whole-foods diet and adding one or two fruit and vegetable juices to your daily routine will go a long way toward flushing your systems and tissues.

Table 10-2 lists some juice and smoothie combinations and the organs they target. Combine three or four fruits and/or vegetables with ½ teaspoon dried herb in a juice or smoothie and vary the combinations each time. Use these detoxifying juices in a daily juicing program or in a specific detoxifying program like the one outlined later in this chapter.

Table 10-2	Detoxifying and Cleansing Combinations		
Juice or Smoothie	*Fruits*	*Vegetables*	*Herbs*
Kidney Flush	Apple, cranberry, grape, lemon, melon, papaya, strawberry, watermelon	Asparagus, beet-root and greens, cabbage, celery, cucumber	Dandelion root, corn silk
Liver Cleanse	Apple, grape, lemon, lime, orange, papaya, pear	Beetroot and greens, carrot, celery, endive, kale, kohlrabi, parsnip, spinach, tomato, turnip root and greens, wheatgrass	Burdock root, dandelion root and leaves, milk thistle, yellow dock root
Bladder Support	Cranberry, melon, pear, watermelon	Beetroot and greens, cabbage, carrot, parsnip, tomato, turnip and greens, wheatgrass	Dandelion leaves, purs-lane, fenugreek
Constipation Support	Apple, blueberry, citrus fruit, elder-berry, melon, papaya, peach, pear, strawberry, watermelon	Cabbage, endive, spinach, wheat-grass	Licorice root, yellow dock root, psyllium seeds

Juice or Smoothie	Fruits	Vegetables	Herbs
Fluid Retention Support	Strawberry, watermelon	Bean sprouts, cucumber	
Intestinal Cleanse	Peach		
Skin and Lymph System Cleanse	Cranberry, grapefruit, lemon, lime, melon, orange, watermelon	Asparagus, beetroot and greens, carrot, cucumber, kohlrabi, bell peppers, Swiss chard, turnip, kohlrabi, wheatgrass	Burdock root, dandelion leaves, Echinacea, fenugreek, parsley

Detoxifying: Two plans

In this section, I outline two detox blueprints for you: a 5-day and a 28-day plan. If you've never cleansed or undergone a detox program, start with a one- or two-day juice fast (see "Juice fasting, step by step," earlier in this chapter) and see how you feel afterward. If you prepare mentally and set aside the time for juice fasting, it will introduce you to the amazing effects of working with your body to allow it to come back into balance.

When you know what to expect from a cleansing program, you can move on to a longer detox period. If you cleanse regularly, you may want to try the five-day plan. The 28-day plan gives your body deep cleansing and detoxing so that your digestive system can be reset and rid of poisons, waste, and sludge.

The longer you stick to a detox plan, the more waste and poisons will be eliminated. If you've been on antibiotics or smoked for a long time, your body will benefit from a longer detox program.

When it comes to detoxing, the important things to remember are the following:

✔ There is no rush to detox. Your body has already started to heal if you've added fresh raw juices and smoothies to your daily diet.

✔ It's just as important to establish clean, healthy food habits as it is to detox. In fact, detoxing comes as one of the last steps in the move toward a healthy existence.

✔ For your mental well-being, you need to start slowly and add challenges as you master each small step so that by the time you're ready to detox, you're sure to complete the program.

Start slowly and find your happy balance, which may only ever be two or three days of cleansing or detoxing.

When you're detoxing, you may experience runny nose, nausea, sore throat, diarrhea, acne, bad breath, or mild fever as the poisons are drawn out and take one last swing. These minor irritations will pass in a day or two, so stay the course and let your body regenerate and reset itself.

Just as with cleansing, you can use dry-brush techniques before your morning showers, warm water enemas, and baking soda/lemon soaking baths to help your body rid itself of toxins (see "During the fast," earlier in this chapter). Light exercise is essential because it helps the lungs and circulatory systems clear themselves.

Check Table 10-2 and be sure to have at least two herbs on hand to add to juices and smoothies. Milk thistle is particularly helpful in breaking down fats in the liver. Probiotic yogurt with *Lactobacillus acidophilus* and *bifidus* bacteria helps to replace digestive bacteria in the gut and is essential if you've recently been taking antibiotic drugs. One cup of probiotic yogurt, three times a day for the five days, is appropriate.

A five-day detoxifying plan

In this section, I outline a five-day detoxifying plan, step by step.

The week before the detox

A good detox deserves a good refrigerator, pantry, and cupboard cleanse. You can't eat what isn't in your kitchen, so keep only foods that are fresh, whole, and organic. Junk, processed, and refined foods are the very foods that are poisoning you, so clear them out of your house at the beginning of your detox plan.

Start doing the following — and continue these steps throughout the entire detox:

✔ Do at least 30 minutes of light exercise throughout the entire detox. Stretching, yoga, walking, dancing, swimming, or playing a non-competitive sport are good for breathing, stretching, and relaxing. The goal here is to help flush poisons through the lungs, muscles, and lymph system.

✔ Eat only organic fruits, vegetables, whole grains, nuts, seeds, probiotic yogurt, chicken, and fish.

✔ Drink eight cups of water every day. Add the juice of half a lemon to each glass because lemon helps to stimulate liver function.

✔ Stay on all medications throughout the detox. Be sure to check with your healthcare provider about going on a detoxification plan.

✔ Eliminate alcohol, caffeine, nicotine, salt, and any recreational drugs.

✔ Eliminate sugar and refined foods (for example, candy, cake, crackers, sodas, white bread, pasta and other wheat products, all dairy products except probiotic yogurt, and all non-organic soy products).

✔ Eliminate junk and fried foods (for example, food in bags, boxes, jars, or tins; packaged, salted, or preserved meats, pickles, condiments, or processed cheese; frozen foods; and all fried foods).

During the detox

Continue the habits you started the week before the detox.

You can make fresh, raw salads, eat raw nuts and seeds, drink herbal teas, and have legumes and whole grains (such as amaranth, brown rice, and quinoa) when indicated in the plan each day — usually at noon or for dinner. Recipes for detox dressing and tea are in the nearby sidebar, "Detox recipes."

When a juice or smoothie is indicated, refer to Table 10-2. For example, on Day 1, you're told to drink a Constipation Support fruit or vegetable smoothie. So, you can make a smoothie made from three or four of the ingredients listed under the Fruits and/or Vegetables column.

Lightening up while detoxing

Throughout the detox, you can eat salads with a dressing made of the following ingredients:

✔ ⅓ cup avocado or nut oil

✔ 2 tablespoons freshly squeezed lemon or lime juice

✔ ½ teaspoon ground ginger

✔ ¼ teaspoon ground cayenne pepper

Just combine all the ingredients in a jar, cap with a tight-fitting lid, and shake the contents until they're well blended.

You can also enjoy a detox tea made of the following ingredients:

✔ 4 parts dried, finely chopped dandelion root

✔ 4 parts dried, finely chopped burdock root

✔ 2 parts dried crushed fenugreek seeds

✔ 1 part dried crushed milk thistle seeds

✔ 4 parts ground licorice root

In a bowl, combine the herbs and mix well. Transfer to a dark glass jar with tight-fitting lid and store in a dry cupboard. When you're ready to make the tea: For every cup, allow 1 teaspoon of tea blend. Add to a teapot and cover with boiling water. Cover the teapot with a lid and steep for ten minutes. Sweeten with honey if desired.

Drink eight glasses of lemon water throughout the day every day.

Day 1

- **Morning:** Drink a Constipation Support fruit or vegetable smoothie. Eat a bowl of old-fashioned oatmeal with fresh fruit.

- **Midmorning:** Drink a Kidney Flush fruit juice.

- **Lunch:** Eat a salad of fresh, raw vegetables with the detox dressing (see the "Detox recipes" sidebar) and whole grains if desired.

- **Midafternoon:** Drink a Liver Cleanse vegetable juice.

- **Dinner:** Eat grilled or steamed fish, a bean salad with detox dressing, and steamed or raw vegetables or grains.

- **Early evening:** Drink a Constipation Support vegetable smoothie.

Day 2

- **Morning:** Drink a Constipation Support fruit or vegetable smoothie. Eat a bowl of fresh fruit.

- **Midmorning:** Drink a Liver Cleanse fruit juice.

- **Lunch:** Drink a Skin and Lymph System Cleanse vegetable juice.

- **Midafternoon:** Drink a Kidney Flush vegetable juice.

- **Dinner:** Eat a bean salad with detox dressing and steamed or raw vegetables or grains.

- **Early evening:** Drink a Constipation Support vegetable smoothie.

Day 3

- **Morning:** Drink a glass of warm water with the juice of ½ lemon. Eat a bowl of fresh fruit.

- **Midmorning:** Drink a Kidney Flush fruit juice.

- **Lunch:** Drink a Skin and Lymph System Cleanse vegetable juice.

- **Midafternoon:** Drink a Liver Cleanse vegetable juice.

- **Dinner:** Drink a Bladder Support vegetable juice.

- **Early evening:** Drink a cup of detox tea (see the "Detox recipes" sidebar).

Day 4

- **Morning:** Drink a Constipation Support fruit or vegetable smoothie. Eat a bowl of fresh fruit.

✔ **Midmorning:** Drink a Liver Cleanse fruit juice.

✔ **Lunch:** Drink a Skin and Lymph System Cleanse vegetable juice.

✔ **Midafternoon:** Drink a Kidney Flush vegetable juice.

✔ **Dinner:** Eat a bean salad with detox dressing and steamed or raw vegetables or grains.

✔ **Early evening:** Drink a Constipation Support vegetable smoothie.

Day 5

✔ **Morning:** Drink a Constipation Support fruit or vegetable smoothie. Eat a bowl of old-fashioned oatmeal with fresh fruit.

✔ **Midmorning:** Drink a Kidney Flush fruit juice.

✔ **Lunch:** Eat a salad of fresh, raw vegetables with detox dressing and whole grains if desired.

✔ **Midafternoon:** Drink a Liver Cleanse vegetable juice.

✔ **Dinner:** Eat grilled or steamed fish, a bean salad with detox dressing, and steamed or raw vegetables or grains.

✔ **Early evening:** Drink a Constipation Support vegetable smoothie.

After the detox

After five days of a coordinated effort to rid yourself of some pretty nasty chemicals, you'll feel clearheaded, leaner, and perhaps a bit lightheaded. Go slowly, adding whole foods by gently expanding the foods you had on Day 5.

A 28-day detoxifying plan

Why would you want to put yourself on a four-week restricted detox plan? Maybe you've experienced the juice high from juice fasting or detoxing for shorter periods of time, and you're emotionally, physically, and mentally ready for a full-on deep-tissue detox. Maybe you saw the benefits of the five-day detoxifying plan and you know that all it takes is about 28 days to change a habit, so you figure the longer detox will help you permanently change to healthy eating habits. If you've experienced long-term toxicity levels, you know that it takes a long-term approach to rid yourself of the chemicals that are interfering with your autoimmune responses or other similar conditions.

Whatever the reasons, the extended plan is still flexible enough to meet your individual needs. It's based around seven days that are repeated four times. Although it looks simple, there are actually a whole range of raw soups and salads that you can make that include lentils; beans; ancient grains; black, red, or brown rice; other whole grains; nuts; seeds; and a wide variety of fruits and vegetables.

Max Tomlinson's *Clean Up Your Diet: The Pure Food Program to Cleanse, Energize, and Revitalize* (Duncan Baird) is an excellent book that provides several programs and recipes based on a whole-foods diet.

This plan is designed to give you three days of juice fasting and four days of very light meals. You should feel lean and light, but if you're hungry, drink a vegetable juice. Try not to eat or snack on solid foods on days 3, 4, and 5.

Drink eight glasses of lemon water throughout the day every day.

Day 1

- **Morning:** Drink a Constipation Support fruit or vegetable smoothie. Eat a bowl of old-fashioned oatmeal with fresh fruit.

- **Midmorning:** Drink a Kidney Flush fruit juice.

- **Lunch:** Eat a salad of fresh, raw vegetables with detox dressing and whole grains if desired.

- **Midafternoon:** Drink a Liver Cleanse vegetable juice.

- **Dinner:** Eat grilled or steamed fish, a bean salad with detox dressing, and steamed or raw vegetables or grains.

- **Early evening:** Drink a Constipation Support vegetable smoothie.

Day 2

- **Morning:** Drink a Constipation Support fruit or vegetable smoothie. Eat a bowl of fresh fruit.

- **Midmorning:** Drink a Liver Cleanse fruit juice.

- **Lunch:** Drink a Skin and Lymph System Cleanse vegetable juice.

- **Midafternoon:** Drink a Kidney Flush vegetable juice.

- **Dinner:** Eat a bean salad with detox dressing and steamed or raw vegetables or grains.

- **Early evening:** Drink a Constipation Support vegetable smoothie.

Day 3

- **Morning:** Drink a glass of warm water with the juice of ½ lemon. Eat a bowl of fresh fruit.

- **Midmorning:** Drink a Kidney Flush fruit juice.

- **Lunch:** Drink a Skin and Lymph System Cleanse vegetable juice.

- **Midafternoon:** Drink a Liver Cleanse vegetable juice.

- **Dinner:** Drink a Bladder Support vegetable juice.

- **Early evening:** Drink a cup of detox tea.

Day 4

- ✔ **Morning:** Drink a glass of warm water with the juice of ½ lemon. Eat a bowl of fresh fruit.

- ✔ **Midmorning:** Drink a Liver Cleanse fruit juice.

- ✔ **Lunch:** Drink a Skin and Lymph System Cleanse vegetable juice.

- ✔ **Midafternoon:** Drink a Kidney Flush vegetable juice.

- ✔ **Dinner:** Drink a Bladder Support vegetable juice.

- ✔ **Early evening:** Drink a cup of detox tea.

Day 5

- ✔ **Morning:** Drink a glass of warm water with the juice of ½ lemon. Eat a bowl of fresh fruit.

- ✔ **Midmorning:** Drink a Kidney Flush fruit juice.

- ✔ **Lunch:** Drink a Skin and Lymph System Cleanse vegetable juice.

- ✔ **Midafternoon:** Drink a Liver Cleanse vegetable juice.

- ✔ **Dinner:** Drink a Bladder Support vegetable juice.

- ✔ **Early evening:** Drink a cup of detox tea.

Changing your environment to reduce toxins

The whole point of cleansing and detoxing is to rid your body of chemicals and wastes that have been stored in organs and tissues. After you've cleaned up your diet, the rational next step is to reduce toxins in your environment. You can do that by

- ✔ Using nontoxic cleaning alternatives at home and in the office wherever possible

- ✔ Choosing natural fibers (wood, metal, and glass) over plastics and synthetic materials for home furnishings

- ✔ Removing from your home any curtains, flooring, rugs, or toys that are made from polyvinyl chloride (PVC)

- ✔ Not using aerosol sprays for cleaners, foods, or cosmetics

- ✔ Finding natural alternatives for toxic materials (for example, white vinegar for window and glass cleaning or castor or mineral oils in place of synthetic lubricants with solvents)

- ✔ Choosing water-based latex paints instead of lead-based paints

- ✔ Having your furnace, fireplace, or gas heater checked regularly to prevent leaks of deadly fumes

Greenpeace has a great website that offers lots of tips on living a green life-style: www.greenpeace.org/usa/en/multimedia/goodies/green-guide/green-lifestyle. It's not a stretch to go from cleaning up your own body to cleaning up the earth.

Day 6

- ✔ **Morning:** Drink a Constipation Support fruit or vegetable smoothie. Eat a bowl of fresh fruit.

- ✔ **Midmorning:** Drink a Liver Cleanse fruit juice.

- ✔ **Lunch:** Drink a Skin and Lymph System Cleanse vegetable juice.

- ✔ **Midafternoon:** Drink a Kidney Flush vegetable juice.

- ✔ **Dinner:** Eat a bean salad with detox dressing and steamed or raw vegetables or grains.

- ✔ **Early evening:** Drink a Constipation Support vegetable smoothie.

Day 7

- ✔ **Morning:** Drink a Constipation Support fruit or vegetable smoothie. Eat a bowl of old-fashioned oatmeal with fresh fruit.

- ✔ **Midmorning:** Drink a Kidney Flush fruit juice.

- ✔ **Lunch:** Eat a salad of fresh, raw vegetables with detox dressing and whole grains if desired.

- ✔ **Midafternoon:** Drink a Liver Cleanse vegetable juice.

- ✔ **Dinner:** Eat grilled or steamed fish, a bean salad with detox dressing, and steamed or raw vegetables or grains.

- ✔ **Early evening:** Drink a Constipation Support vegetable smoothie.

Trying Some Detox Drinks

Detoxing means that you're serious about cleansing and clearing out not only toxins, but also old habits. In this section, I detail some detox drinks to get you started on your way to a lighter, more enlightened existence.

Feeling good is only a detox away. It may seem that it gets worse — and it may, but for only a few days — and then it gets better . . . a lot better. First, you'll feel like a veil has lifted in your brain. You loose the fuzzy feeling and begin to think clearly. You can make decisions and actually feel alive, and then you realize that your normal state isn't your optimal state.

In fact, your optimal state is one in which you handle problems and stress with grace and you solve problems calmly. Detoxing may also relieve the following symptoms:

✔ Bloating

✔ Dark circles, puffy eyes, or bags under or above your eyes

✔ Fatigue

✔ Low-grade infections

✔ Many allergies

✔ Rash, acne, or irritated skin

✔ Sluggishness

Antiox-Detox

Prep time: About 2 min • **Juicing time:** 2min • **Yield:** 2 small servings

Ingredients	Directions
1 cup blue or blackberries	*1* Turn on the juicer and place a jug under the spout.
2 black plums, halved and stoned	*2* Working on a slow speed, process the berries, plums, and fresh cranberries.
½ cup fresh or frozen (thawed) cranberries	
1 wedge red cabbage	*3* Increase the speed to medium and process the cranberries if frozen, the cabbage, and the fresh dandelion root, if using.
1-inch piece fresh dandelion root or 1 teaspoon powdered dried dandelion root	
1 tablespoon pure maple syrup or coconut nectar	*4* Stir the powdered dried dandelion root if fresh isn't available, and the maple syrup into the juice in the jug. Pour into 2 glasses and enjoy!

Per serving: Calories 126 (From Fat 3); Fat 0g (Saturated 0g); Cholesterol 0mg; Sodium 12mg; Carbohydrate 33g (Dietary Fiber 1g); Protein 2g.

Tip: For juicing, when a wedge of cabbage or melon is called for, the vegetable or fruit is cut into quarters and each quarter is cut in half (or smaller) so that the wedge will fit into the tube of the juicer lid. If you want to use two wedges of cabbage in this recipe because of its antioxidant benefits, go right ahead.

Loving Your Liver Detox

Prep time: About 2 min • **Juicing time:** 2 min • **Yield:** 2 small servings

Ingredients	Directions
4 kale leaves	*1* Wash and pat kale leaves dry, leaving on the stalk. Wash and quarter the beets.
2 carrots	
1 apple	*2* Turn on the juicer and place a jug under the spout.
1-inch piece fresh gingerroot	
2 beets	*3* Working on a slow speed, process the kale leaves.
½ teaspoon powdered milk thistle	*4* Increase the speed to medium and process the carrots and apple.
	5 Increase the speed to high and process the gingerroot and beets.
	6 Stir the powdered milk thistle into the juice in the jug, pour into 2 glasses and enjoy!

Per serving: Calories 131 (From Fat 6); Fat 1g (Saturated 0g); Cholesterol 0mg; Sodium 138mg; Carbohydrate 31g (Dietary Fiber 2g); Protein 4g.

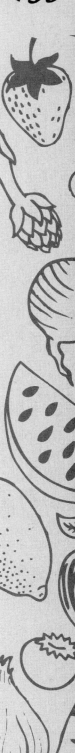

Tropical Ade

Prep time: About 3 min • **Juicing time:** 2 min • **Yield:** 2 servings

Ingredients	Directions
2 oranges, peeled with pith intact	*1* Turn on the juicer and place a jug under the spout.
1 mango, peeled and seeded 1 grapefruit, peeled with pith intact	*2* Working on a slow speed, process the oranges, mango, and grapefruit.
1-inch piece fresh burdock root or 2 teaspoons powdered dried burdock root	*3* Increase speed to medium and process the fresh burdock root and carrots.
2 carrots	*4* If using powdered dried burdock root, stir it into the juice in the jug. Pour into 2 glasses and enjoy!

Per serving: Calories 232 (From Fat 5); Fat 1g (Saturated 0g); Cholesterol 0mg; Sodium 60mg; Carbohydrate 56g (Dietary Fiber 3g); Protein 3g.

Tip: Burdock root is very effective as a gentle cleanser and is worth the effort to find it. Sometimes Asian grocery stores sell the fresh root in the spring and fall, otherwise look for the dried powdered root in natural food stores. If you can't find bulk powdered herbs, you can break open gel capsules to add herbs to juices or smoothies.

Part III
Juicing to Your Heart's Desire

The nitty-gritty of juicing

- Fresh, raw fruit and vegetables are packed with vitamins, phytochemicals, and fiber that have been proven to protect against disease.

- Drinking at least one fresh vegetable or fruit juice every day adds from three to five servings of these powerful ingredients.

- Due to their lower natural sugars, vegetable juice is the preferred drink of people who optimize their healthy drinks.

- Adding the pulp from juicing to smoothies, baked products, soups, and other recipes, increases their fiber and nutrient content.

Head to www.dummies.com/extras/juicingsmoothies for some tips and suggestions for cooking with fresh, homemade juice.

In this part . . .

- ✔ Get started with juicing ingredients and tips. When you know what you can and can't juice and how to use juices in lots of different recipes, you'll be raring to go.

- ✔ Begin making your own juices with dozens of juice recipes — for both fruit and vegetable juices.

- ✔ Create juices for any time of the day — breakfast, lunch, dinner, and snacks — that are tasty and nutritious.

- ✔ Be creative and know what to do and how to use your juicing leftovers.

Chapter 11

Identifying Juice Ingredients and Techniques

....

In This Chapter

▶ Stocking up on ingredients for juicing

▶ Mastering the juicing technique

▶ Cooking with juices

....

I know what it's like to bring the juicer home and take it out of the box for the first time. You're probably excited and a bit nervous. If so, you've come to the right chapter. Here, I start out by telling you what to look for in terms of juicing ingredients. Then I explain how to make juices — there's nothing to be intimidated by, trust me. Finally, I close the chapter by telling you how you can use those fabulous juices you've made in a variety of dishes — everything from sauces to soups and more! If you're new to the world of juicing, this chapter will help you start your juicing journey on the right foot.

Naming Common Juicing Ingredients

Fruit, vegetables, herbs, sprouts, and grasses — that's the extent of ingredients that you can juice. In this section, I walk you through the wide variety of ingredients that fall into these categories. I also show you some healthy ingredients you can add to juices. (For more information on shopping for fresh produce, check out Chapter 4.)

Fruits and vegetables

Nature has conveniently color-coded the major phytonutrients into four major shades — orange/yellow, red, blue/purple, and green — and each is brimming with healthy components. Spread your 9 to 12 servings of fruits and vegetables among the four color groups, and you're guaranteed to be following the best possible diet for good health.

Orange/yellow

Alpha- and beta-carotene, lutein, and lycopene are the biological pigments that give orange/yellow fruits and vegetables their color. Studies show that orange/yellow plant foods protect against cancer and stroke. Eating one or two every day will guard against heart disease, cancer, and other modern ailments.

What you can't juice

A juicing machine or juice extractor removes the juice or liquid from fruits or vegetables by force. And because the machine is doing the squeezing and separating of the pulp and juice, you can juice many hard fruits and vegetables that you couldn't juice by hand. Still, there are a few fruits and vegetables that simply can't be forced into giving up their precious liquids. You can use these fruits and vegetables in smoothies but not in juices:

✔ **Avocado:** Avocado is a great source of omega-3 fatty acids and, when ripe, it blends nicely, making smoothies and dips creamy and smooth. But if you try to juice it, it will only jam your juice machine. You can add avocado to fresh juice, though — here's how: In a blender, combine 1 cup fresh juice with ½ avocado, cut into chunks. Blend until smooth. Pour this mixture into the rest of your juice and mix well. The avocado will make the juice thick and creamy.

✔ **Banana:** Bananas are high in potassium, but they gum up the working parts of the juicer when you try to juice them. To add bananas to your glass of fresh juice, follow these steps: In a blender, combine 1 cup fresh juice with ½ banana, cut into chunks.

Blend until smooth. Pour this mixture into the rest of your juice and mix well.

✔ **Rhubarb:** Rhubarb leaves are high in oxalic acid and inedible, but the stalks contain such tiny amounts of the toxic acid that most people can eat small amounts of rhubarb stalks in pie and jam without experiencing problems. However, because of the amount of fresh rhubarb required to make one glass of juice, the amount of nutrients and the toxic oxalic acid is concentrated and much higher than if you eat the stalks raw. Juicing rhubarb could cause a reaction of stomach irritation and kidney problems, so you're better off leaving it for smoothies and rhubarb pie.

✔ **Winter squash:** Winter squash is just too hard to juice. In fact, you can damage your grating basket or blades if you try to juice raw squash. But the nutrients are exceptional, so to juice squash, you can soften chunks of butternut or acorn squash by lightly steaming them before juicing.

✔ **Nuts, seeds, and grains:** Nuts, seeds, and grains aren't suitable for juicing, but you can finely chop them and add them to fresh juice as a protein boost.

Here are some great examples of orange/yellow fruits and vegetables you can juice:

- ✔ Apricots
- ✔ Bell peppers
- ✔ Cantaloupe
- ✔ Carrots
- ✔ Grapefruit
- ✔ Lemons
- ✔ Mangoes
- ✔ Nectarines
- ✔ Oranges

- ✔ Papayas
- ✔ Peaches
- ✔ Pineapple
- ✔ Plums
- ✔ Pumpkin
- ✔ Squash
- ✔ Sweet potatoes
- ✔ Tangerines
- ✔ Yams

Red

Seven of the top 20 antioxidant fruits and vegetables are red. *Anthocyanins* (the bright red, purple, and blue pigments found in plants), cancer-fighting ellagic acid, and vitamin C, among other things, are high in this color group. Just like the heat and emotion they represent, red fruits and vegetables are essential to the daily diet, so plan to include one or two of these balls of fire in your daily juice or smoothie regimen.

Here are some examples of red fruits and vegetables you can juice:

- ✔ Apples
- ✔ Beets
- ✔ Bell peppers
- ✔ Cherries
- ✔ Cranberries
- ✔ Plums

- ✔ Pomegranates
- ✔ Raspberries
- ✔ Red onions
- ✔ Grapes
- ✔ Strawberries
- ✔ Tomatoes

Blue/purple

Bright blue/purple vegetables get their pigment from anthocyanins and beta-carotene, both excellent cancer-fighters. Aim to include one blue-purple fruit or vegetable every day.

Here are some examples of blue/purple fruits and vegetables you can juice:

- Bilberries
- Blackberries
- Blueberries
- Concord grapes
- Eggplants

- Elderberries
- Purple carrots
- Purple potatoes
- Purple tomatoes

Green

Chlorophyll is the pigment that gives green fruits and vegetables their color. Green foods are good sources of carotenoids (vitamin A precursors), including lutein and powerful antioxidants. Green vegetables tend to score lower on the glycemic index chart (see Chapter 5 for more on the glycemic index), so they're a good balancing addition to juices.

Juice the following green vegetables in small amounts once you're enjoying a wide variety of new vegetables:

- Asparagus
- Bell peppers
- Broccoli
- Brussels sprouts
- Cabbage
- Collard greens

- Kale
- Musk melon
- Mustard greens
- Spinach
- Swiss chard

Dark green vegetables are powerful laxatives. Start with a ratio of one dark green vegetable to four to six other vegetables, and don't introduce dark green vegetables until you've enjoyed a wide variety of new vegetable colors and tastes because they're strong and potent.

Green grasses, herbs, and sprouts

Cereal grasses (from barley, rye, buckwheat, and wheat) and sprouts (from beans and lentils) are nutrition powerhouses because they contain all the nutrients necessary for growing the mature plant. Wild weeds and cultivated herbs offer a wide range of vitamins, minerals, and phytonutrients, with chlorophyll as an added bonus. Use them fresh, or whisk powdered greens (available at natural food stores) into juices.

If you're interested in growing your own grasses and herbs and sprouting your own seeds so that the nutrients are at their peak when you juice them, check out *Container Gardening For Dummies,* 2nd Edition, by Bill Marken, Suzanne DeJohn, and the Editors of the National Gardening Association (Wiley).

 Not every juicing machine can efficiently extract juice from grasses, herbs, and sprouts, so if you're buying a juicing machine, look for one that can handle these delicate sprigs. If you already own a good juicer but want to enjoy juices from grasses, herbs, and sprouts, look for one of a few inexpensive and hand-turned, strictly grass juicers.

Here are some of the edible grasses, herbs, and sprouts to add to fruit or vegetable juice for the benefits they bring:

- Alfalfa sprouts
- Barley greens
- Buckwheat greens
- Lentil sprouts
- Parsley (***Note:*** Pregnant women and people with kidney problems should avoid parsley juice.)
- Purslane
- Watercress
- Wheatgrass

Healthy additives

If you're anything like me, you'll end up mostly taking your juices straight — with no ice, and with nothing stirred, shaken, or whisked in. But every once in a while, you may want to add some super healthy ingredient to your juices, and that's why this section is important.

Don't overload your juices with extra stuff. Instead, choose one additive from one or two of the following groups per glass of juice.

- **Group 1:** Nuts, seeds, and parts or the wheat kernel

  - **Bran:** Add 1 tablespoon of ground oat bran or wheat bran per glass of juice.

  - **Chia seeds:** A complete protein and gluten-free food with a high antioxidant level as well as a rich source of omega-3 fatty acids, chia seeds are a great juice additive. Soak a teaspoon of the seeds in juice or water for about 10 minutes and stir into a glass of freshly processed juice. The juice will be thick because chia absorbs up to 10 times its weight.

- **Flaxseed:** Whole flaxseeds pass through the body virtually intact without releasing their nutrients and fats, so you want to make sure to use ground flaxseed. Flaxseed contains alpha linolenic acid (ALA), which the body uses to produce omega-3 fatty acids. Add a tablespoon ground flaxseed per glass of juice.

- **Hemp:** In many places, hemp seeds are illegal (because of their connection to marijuana), but they're a great source of protein, fiber, and omega-6 and omega-3 fatty acids. Start with 1 teaspoon and work up to 1 tablespoon of hemp seeds in juice daily. If hemp seeds are unavailable, use wheat germ and up to 1 tablespoon of hemp oil.

- **Wheat germ:** The *germ* is the tiny core of the grain. It contains nutrients for the plant. Two tablespoons deliver 4 grams of protein, 2 grams of fiber, and about 1.5 grams of unsaturated fat. Add 1 tablespoon wheat germ per glass of juice.

✔ **Group 2:** Herbs and spices

- **Basil:** Basil is calming and works as an antidepressant when used in medicinal quantities. For juicing, use three to six fresh leaves of basic, or whisk in ¼ teaspoon fresh chopped leaves to each glass of juice.

- **Cinnamon:** Cinnamon can help moderate blood sugar, which is good news for diabetics and people who are weight-conscious. Cinnamon is an antioxidant and inhibits ulcers, as well as being helpful in reducing joint pain and muscle stiffness. Add ¼ teaspoon of ground cinnamon per glass of juice.

- **Dandelion:** The leaves of this common plant are high in vitamins C and K, and they're also a tonic for the liver and gallbladder, helping to excrete toxins.

- **Garlic:** Garlic's antioxidant, antibacterial, heart-protecting, and anti-cancer properties give it healing power. Juice one peeled clove of garlic for each serving of juice.

- **Ginger:** I use ginger to treat headaches, nausea, and vomiting, but ginger has anti-inflammatory and antioxidant properties, so you may want to add it to drinks often. Use ¼ teaspoon freshly grated raw ginger or a pinch of ground ginger per serving of juice.

- **Licorice:** Well known as a soothing throat and stomach medicine, licorice supports the immune system. It also has anti-inflammatory and anti-tumor properties. Use ¼ teaspoon ground licorice root per juice serving.

- **Oregano:** With its powerful antioxidants and minerals — including magnesium, zinc, potassium, iron, boron, and manganese — as well as vitamins A and C, oregano is an important healing herb. Add ¼ teaspoon of finely chopped fresh leaves (or a pinch dried) per serving of juice.

- **Rosemary:** Use rosemary in small amounts (1 fresh sprig juiced with grasses or a pinch freshly chopped) for a zing of fresh citrus-menthol flavor and lots of chlorophyll.

- **Thyme:** I grow and use thyme in cooking because of its antioxidants. Use ¼ teaspoon finely chopped fresh thyme leaves per juice serving.

- **Turmeric:** The anti-inflammatory properties of turmeric help alleviate arthritis and joint pain, so add it to juices after exercising. Turmeric also fights tumors and is an antioxidant. Blend ¼ teaspoon of ground turmeric per juice serving.

✔ **Group 3:** Natural super supplements

- **Bee pollen:** Bee pollen is loaded with vitamins, amino acids, minerals, trace elements, and enzymes. Start by grinding bee pollen in a blender and then whisk ½ teaspoon into a glass of juice.

- **Brewer's yeast:** As a rich source of the B-complex vitamins and with essential amino acids and minerals including chromium, brewer's yeast is a good natural supplement. Stir ¼ teaspoon of powder into a glass of juice.

- **Propolis:** Bees mix a resinous sap from trees with wax and use it for general hive maintenance; this sap is called propolis. With its ability to fight infection and its antimicrobial, antioxidant, anti-ulcer, and antitumor qualities, propolis is great for humans, too. Whisk ½ teaspoon into a glass of juice.

- **Umeboshi:** A paste made from pickled plums, this Asian health food is valued for its antibacterial and pH balancing effect. Best of all, it's used to curb sugar addiction and cravings. Whisk in ½ teaspoon per juice serving.

✔ **Group 4:** Tinctures, tonics, and elixirs

- **Tinctures:** The whole or specific parts of an herb are immersed in alcohol to extract their active components. Tinctures are available in whole-food or health food stores. Some tincture herbs are astragalus and echinacea for immune boosting; valerian and hops to calm nerves; dandelion and milk thistle to cleanse; and ginseng and mint to refresh and stimulate. You can add tinctures by the drop to juices. Follow guidelines for doses given by the manufacturer or a qualified herbalist.

- **Tonic teas:** Tonic herbs are considered superior because they strengthen the body and prevent illness (as opposed to medicinal or inferior herbs, which treat illness). Tonic herbs such as parsley, basil, and stinging nettles balance and nourish; ginseng, astragalus, and licorice help the body to adjust to stress, aging, and pollutants. Whisk up to ¼ cup of a tonic tea into a glass of juice.

- **Elixirs:** Teas or whole herb liquid extractions made from tonic herbs often are combined with natural, healthy supplements like those listed in Group 3. These drinks are called elixirs. Juices made with antioxidant fruits and/or vegetables that also include a tonic tea or tincture are great-tasting elixirs.

Taking Note of Juicing Techniques

Juicing can be a part of your diet for life if you build healthy habits. If your diet is already filled with 9 to 12 servings of fresh fruits and vegetables in a day, you'll be able to move into a juicing regime fairly quickly. However, if you're like most people, and you rely on processed foods and a few overcooked vegetables, you'll need to slowly introduce fresh, raw fruits and vegetables into your diet.

Ease into juicing with fruits and milder vegetables like celery, fennel, and cucumber. Gradually add fresh greens like spinach, romaine lettuce, and green and red leaf lettuce. Next, introduce cabbage and other dark leafy greens. Finally, use carrots and beets sparingly because they're high in sugars.

The goal is to move away from all-fruit juices toward all-vegetable juices or a juice combination of mostly vegetables and a few fruits. Because the nutrients in fresh raw juices pass directly through the stomach lining to the blood and the cells, the best time to drink your fresh juice combinations is on an empty stomach — at least 30 minutes before or one hour after meals.

When your cells and digestive tract are flushed with the raw, live, and pure phytonutrients, enzymes, and other nutrients from fresh fruits and vegetables, your body may experience a detox reaction. You may suffer from headaches, fatigue, joint pain, muscle weakness, and/or diarrhea for the first few days after beginning to juice. All these symptoms should pass within a week, leaving you with increased energy and a feeling of overall health and vigor.

In this section, I share some of the ways to make juicing easy and fun for everyone in your family.

If you want to cook with juices, head to www.dummies.com/extras/ juicingsmoothies for more information.

Peeling, seeding, and coring (or not)

All fruits and vegetables need to be washed with either food-safe soap and water or vinegar and water before juicing, but peeling depends on how the plants were grown. If you're using organic fruits and vegetables (which I strongly recommend), don't peel (the skin is good for you if it's organic); if you're using non-organic, peel before juicing.

I leave the cores and seeds intact on fruits and vegetables such as apples, kiwis, watermelons, cucumbers, and summer squash, except if I'm planning to use the pulp to make baked goods or sauces. Because I don't want to include the harder, bitterer tasting core and seeds in products like muffins and quick breads, I core and seed if I plan to save the pulp.

Juicing from soft to hard and using different juicer speeds

If you have a multi-speed juicer, it's easiest on the machine if you start juicing soft fruits and vegetables (like citrus fruits or tomatoes) at the lower speed, and gradually increase the speed as the fruits or vegetables get firmer. You start on low speed because the liquid in a soft fruit or vegetable is easier to extract than that of a hard one.

If you use a slow speed for soft items, you'll extract more juice from them because, at a high speed, they fly right through the blades and much of the juice remains in the pulp. In contrast, for hard vegetables like beets and ruta-baga, you need a higher speed of the blades to cut through the denser flesh, and you need the faster spinning basket to extract the juice from the fiber.

Juicing fresh herbs and grasses

The first time you try to juice cabbage or lettuce leaves, green grasses, or herbs, unless your juicer can handle grasses, you'll find that they jam in the basket and make a mess. Cut cabbage into wedges, and it'll pass through the juicing basket easily.

If you don't want to add too much strong cabbage taste to a juice, but you have a few large outer leaves that you want to combine with other ingredients, the best way to get the most out of the leaves is to roll them into a tight, long cylindrical shape and guide them through the feed tube using celery stalks, carrots, or apple wedges.

Herb sprigs and cereal grasses are more delicate and more difficult to juice without the benefit of a special attachment. If you wedge a handful of green grasses or herbs in the natural groove of a celery stalk and use a slow speed, the celery will keep the grass in place long enough for the juice to be extracted.

You also can "juice" wheatgrass and herbs using a blender. This method is more efficient in extracting the essential and active elements in wheatgrass. Here's how to do it:

1. **In the blender container, combine 1½ cups water with 2 to 3 cups of fresh wheatgrass.**

2. **Process the mixture on high for 30 to 40 seconds or until the grass is liquefied.**

3. **Line a sieve with a layer of cheesecloth and set it over a large bowl.**

4. **Pour the wheatgrass and water through the sieve into the bowl.**

5. **Squeeze the cheesecloth to remove all the moisture from the wheatgrass.**

6. **Blend ¼ to ½ of the wheatgrass juice into fresh fruit or vegetable juice.**

Chapter 12

Making Some Easy Fruit Juices

. . . .

In This Chapter

▶ Starting off your day with breakfast

▶ Taking a break with a snack

▶ Boosting digestion and your immune system

▶ Getting the party started with fruit mocktails, cocktail mixers, and punches

. . . .

Drinking fruit juices for breakfast and for early morning snacks gives you energy in the form of fructose (fruit sugar). And fructose is released slowly, which means that it doesn't spike your blood sugar and then leave you feeling deflated the way refined sugar does.

Fruit juices are best taken on their own before protein foods or one to two hours after, so early morning and midmorning are the optimum times for drinking them.

If you suffer from poor digestion, natural fruit juices can help. Some tropical fruits, like pineapples, kiwifruits, and papayas, have super enzymes that help the digestive system do its job. And although these foods actually help your body digest food, herbs like peppermint and dandelion root kickstart your liver and gallbladder and increase the flow of bile so that your organs are more efficient.

I wrap up this chapter with mocktail recipes, because when you start to drink to your health, alcohol is one of the things that you may choose to cut down on or eliminate. The mocktails in this chapter taste so great on their own, there really is no need to add alcohol — but if you want to socialize once in a while, the cocktail mixers and fruit punch recipes offer a tasty way to sneak in a few extra nutrients in place of the empty calories in soda.

WARNING! If you have low blood sugar (hypoglycemia) or are diabetic, consult your doctor before starting to juice fruits. If you have a yeast infection (like thrush or candidiasis), do not drink fruit juice until these problems are resolved.

Starting Your Morning the Right Way: Breakfast Juices

Citrus fruit and orange juice in particular are top-of-the-morning favorites, but you can drink any of the brilliantly hued fruits available fresh and in season. In fact, the brighter the drink, the better! So, break your overnight fast with a big, beautiful, liquid breakfast.

Begin slowly with juicing

I know you want to jump right in with juicing — after all, you're charged up about doing something positive for your health! But rein in your enthusiasm (not for long, just at the beginning) and let your taste buds, digestive system, liver, kidneys, colon, and the rest of your body acclimate to this new and exciting diet.

Here are some tips for tiptoeing into the juice fever:

✔ **Don't underestimate the power of the live enzymes, phytonutrients, and other healthy components in fresh fruit and vegetables.** They pack a punch! Start out with a half-glass (4 ounces) for the first few days, or dilute 4 ounces with water.

✔ **Start with fruit if you don't like the taste of vegetables, and gradually add vegetables while decreasing the fruit.** The ultimate goal is to be juicing more vegetables than fruit in a ratio of about two to one, but this may take a year for you to achieve. Don't rush — enjoy the journey!

✔ **Start with mild vegetables.** Carrot, cucumber, and celery are easy to take at first. You can gradually add stronger-tasting vegetables like spinach, turnip, beets, cabbage, and onions, but try them one at a time.

✔ **Listen to your body.** It will tell you if you need to slow down or if it can handle the amount of fresh, raw juice you're giving it. Even a small amount of raw beet juice, for example, may cause you to experience cramps, gas, and diarrhea. This doesn't mean that you'll never be able to drink beet juice; it just means that your body needs time to get used to it.

✔ **Don't indulge in too much of a good thing.** Straight green juice, for example, may burn your throat if you take it without mixing a small amount in other juices or diluting it with water. Always introduce new ingredients one at a time and in small amounts. See how your body reacts before you gradually increase the amount.

✔ **Stay with it!** In time, your sense of taste will change and your body will enjoy the benefits that a fresh fruit and vegetable regimen brings.

Sunny Side Up

Prep time: About 3 min • **Juicing time:** 2 min • **Yield:** 2 servings

Ingredients	Directions
2 kiwifruits	*1* Peel kiwifruits and guavas.
2 guavas	*2* Peel oranges and lemon, leaving the white pith on.
2 oranges	
1 lemon	*3* Turn on the juicer and place a jug under the spout.
	4 Working on a slow speed, process the kiwifruits, guavas, oranges, and lemon.
	5 Stir the drink, pour into 2 glasses, and enjoy!

Per serving: Calories 164 (From Fat 9); Fat 1g (Saturated 0g); Cholesterol 0mg; Sodium 10mg; Carbohydrate 41g (Dietary Fiber 6g); Protein 3g.

Save the pith

Chefs and cooks have always been pretty clear about removing the white pith that surrounds all citrus fruit because of its bitter flavor. The truth is, there are a lot of nutrients in that bitter white stuff, along with insoluble fiber in the form of pectin. It was by sheer chance that I discovered firsthand that if you carefully cut away the sharply tart and strong, colored rind (called *exocarp*) and leave the white, spongy pith (called *endocarp*) surrounding citrus fruit, somehow when you juice the pith-covered fruit, a creamy, delicious juice is the happy result.

This juice is very different from citrus fruit that's pressed or squeezed for the juice. The juice that is the result of pressing or squeezing or using a reamer (or any device) that forces the delicious liquid out of citrus fruit halves is thin and acidic.

Remember: When juicing any fruit or vegetable with the skin (or in this case, with the layer of tissue so close to the outer rind), it should be organic so herbicides or pesticides don't intrude.

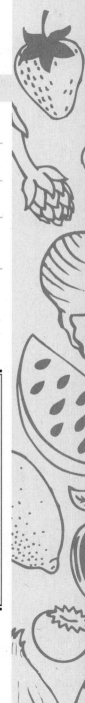

Peaches and Dreams

Prep time: About 15 min • **Juicing time:** 2 min • **Yield:** 1 serving

Ingredients	Directions
2 peaches	**1** Cut the peaches in half and remove the stones.
1 lime	**2** Peel the lime, leaving the white pith on.
2 pomegranates	**3** Break apart each of the pomegranates into 4 pieces (you'll have 8 pieces total) and pull out the red seeds. Discard the rind and the white membrane.
2 pears	**4** Cut the pears if necessary to fit the juicer feed tube.
	5 Turn on the juicer and place a jug under the spout.
	6 Working on a slow speed, process the peaches and lime.
	7 Increase the speed to medium and process the pomegranate seeds and pears.
	8 Stir the drink, pour into 2 glasses, and enjoy!

Per serving: Calories 510 (From Fat 22); Fat 2g (Saturated 0g); Cholesterol 0mg; Sodium 9mg; Carbohydrate 132g (Dietary Fiber 4g); Protein 6g.

Perfect in Pink

Prep time: About 2 min • **Juicing time:** 2 min • **Yield:** 2 servings

Ingredients	Directions
1 cup raspberries	*1* Wash the raspberries and grapes under gently streaming water; pat dry.
½ cup red grapes	
½ lemon	*2* Peel the lemon, leaving the white pith on.
2 slices (1-inch thick) watermelon	*3* Peel and discard the rind and the white part of the watermelon. Cut it into pieces to fit the juicer feed tube.
2 apples	*4* Cut the apples if necessary to fit the juicer feed tube.
	5 Turn on the juicer and place a jug under the spout.
	6 Working on a slow speed, process the raspberries, grapes, lemon, and watermelon.
	7 Stir the drink, pour into 2 glasses, and enjoy!

Per serving: Calories 225 (From Fat 10); Fat 1g (Saturated 0g); Cholesterol 0mg; Sodium 8mg; Carbohydrate 57g (Dietary Fiber 3g); Protein 3g.

Vary It: Try blueberries or cherries in place of the raspberries.

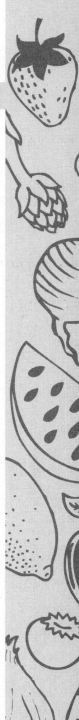

Black Pearl

Prep time: About 2 min • **Juicing time:** 2 min • **Yield:** 1 serving

Ingredients	Directions
2 cups blackberries **1 cup blueberries** **½ lime** **2 nectarines or fresh apricots** **2 black plums**	**1** Wash the blackberries and blueberries under gently streaming water; pat dry.
	2 Peel the lime, leaving the white pith on.
	3 Cut the nectarines and plums in half and remove the stones.
	4 Turn on the juicer and place a jug under the spout.
	5 Working on a slow speed, process the blackberries, blueberries, and lime.
	6 Increase the speed to medium and process the nectarines and plums.
	7 Clean the juicer.
	8 Stir the drink, pour into 2 glasses, and enjoy!

Per serving: Calories 447 (From Fat 34); Fat 4g (Saturated 0g); Cholesterol 0mg; Sodium 9mg; Carbohydrate 110g (Dietary Fiber 8g); Protein 7g.

Ginger Flax Starter

Prep time: About 2 min • **Juicing time:** 2 min • **Yield:** 1 serving

Ingredients	Directions
1 orange	*1* Peel the orange, leaving the white pith intact.
2 nectarines or fresh apricots	
2 cups fresh or frozen (thawed) peach slices	*2* Cut the nectarines in half and remove the stones.
2 medium carrots	*3* Turn on the juicer and place a jug under the spout.
1 piece (1-inch) peeled fresh ginger	*4* Working on a slow speed, process the orange, nectarines, and peach slices.
2 tablespoons ground flaxseed	
	5 Increase speed to medium and process the carrots and ginger.
	6 Stir the flaxseed into the drink, pour into 2 glasses, and enjoy!

Per serving: Calories 426 (From Fat 56); Fat 6g (Saturated 0g); Cholesterol 0mg; Sodium 101mg; Carbohydrate 9g (Dietary Fiber 5g); Protein 11g.

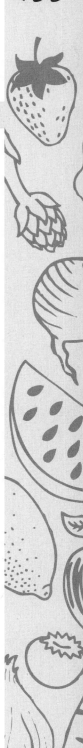

Juicing between Meals: Snack Juices

A glass of fresh juice makes the perfect midmorning or midafternoon snack. It gives a boost of energy when you feel you're running out of steam.

If you double any of the breakfast or snack recipes, you'll have enough to enjoy immediately and to fill a thermos or jar for later.

Storing juice: How long is okay?

You start to really enjoy the taste, the benefits, the energy, and the vitality that juicing can give and you think, "Why not save time and effort by making a day's (or a few days') worth of juice?" Believe me, it's a great idea — and you're not the first person to have it. The only problem is, vitamins B2, B6, E, and, to a degree, C are all sensitive to light. If they're exposed to light when the produce is stored, during juicing, or during the storage of the juice, those vitamins will be lost.

The best possible practice is to drink your juice as soon as possible after it's juiced. That means it isn't a good idea to juice hours before a meal or the night before. Now, my personal view is that if this will be the one thing that will enable you to enjoy fresh, raw, handmade juice, then go for it because any loss of nutrients won't stack up to the incredible benefits you'll still enjoy by consuming fresh juice.

If you really want to store freshly juiced produce, here are some tips to ensure that your precious juice doesn't lose nutrients during storage:

✔ **Store juice in a glass jar with a tight-fitting lid that doesn't allow for a lot of air.** The goal is less than ½ inch of air space between the juice and the lid.

✔ **If possible, the glass jar should be dark to filter out light and UV rays.**

✔ **Refrigerate fresh juice immediately and keep chilled until ready to use.**

✔ **Use within 24 hours.** Bacteria can grow in a liquid like water or juice without preservatives very quickly, even if it's stored in the refrigerator.

Citrus and Mango Tango

Prep time: About 2 min • **Juicing time:** 2 min • **Yield:** 2 servings

Ingredients	Directions
2 oranges	*1* Peel the oranges and grapefruit, leaving the white pith on.
1 ruby red grapefruit	
2 mangos	*2* Peel the mangos and remove the pits.
½ cantaloupe melon	
	3 Scoop out the seeds and trim away the rind from the cantaloupe. Discard the seeds and rind. Cut the cantaloupe flesh into wedges to fit the juicer feed tube.
	4 Turn on the juicer and place a jug under the spout.
	5 Working on a slow speed, process the oranges and grapefruit.
	6 Increase speed to medium and process the mangos and melon.
	7 Stir the drink, pour into 2 glasses, and enjoy!

Per serving: Calories 285 (From Fat 11); Fat 1g (Saturated 0g); Cholesterol 0mg; Sodium 17mg; Carbohydrate 73g (Dietary Fiber 6g); Protein 4g.

Vary It: Try blood oranges when they're in season.

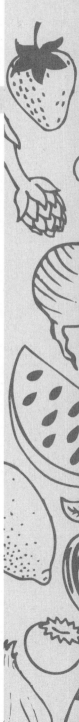

Berries and Cream

Prep time: About 3 min • **Juicing time:** 2 min • **Yield:** 2 servings

Ingredients	Directions
1 cup raspberries	*1* Wash the raspberries under gently streaming water; pat dry.
1 orange	
3 cups cranberries, thawed if frozen	*2* Peel the orange, leaving the white pith on.
1 apple	*3* In a sieve, run the cranberries under hot water to thaw if frozen; pat dry.
1 cup plain or vanilla yogurt	
	4 Cut the apple if necessary to fit the juicer feed tube.
	5 Turn on the juicer and place a jug under the spout.
	6 Working on a slow speed, process the raspberries and orange.
	7 Increase the speed to medium and process the cranberries and apple.
	8 Stir in the yogurt, pour into 2 glasses, and enjoy!

Per serving: *Calories 249 (From Fat 26); Fat 3g (Saturated 1g); Cholesterol 7mg; Sodium 87mg; Carbohydrate 52g (Dietary Fiber 5g); Protein 8g.*

The Daily Double

Prep time: About 2 min • **Juicing time:** 2 min • **Yield:** 2 servings

Ingredients	Directions
1 cup strawberries **4 oranges** **2 apples**	*1* Wash the strawberries under gently streaming water, hull, and pat dry.
	2 Peel the oranges, leaving the white pith on.
	3 Cut the apples if necessary to fit the juicer feed tube.
	4 Turn on the juicer and place a jug under the spout.
	5 Working on a slow speed, process the strawberries and oranges.
	6 Increase the speed to medium and process the apples.
	7 Stir the drink, pour into 2 glasses, and enjoy!

Per serving: Calories 227 (From Fat 10); Fat 1g (Saturated 0g); Cholesterol 0mg; Sodium 1mg; Carbohydrate 57g (Dietary Fiber 6g); Protein 3g.

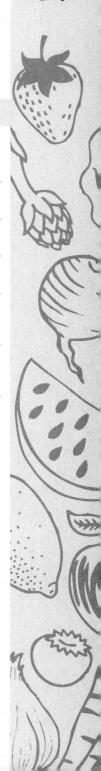

Mint Chiller

Prep time: About 3 min • **Juicing time:** 2 min • **Yield:** 2 servings

Ingredients	Directions
3 kiwifruits	*1* Peel the kiwifruits and oranges, leaving the white pith on the oranges.
2 oranges	
½ muskmelon	*2* Scoop out the seeds and trim away the rind from the melon. Discard the seeds and rind. Cut the melon flesh into wedges to fit the juicer feed tube.
1 piece (1-inch) peeled fresh ginger	
½ to 1 tablespoon finely chopped fresh mint	*3* Turn on the juicer and place a jug under the spout.
	4 Working on a slow speed, process the kiwifruits and oranges.
	5 Increase the speed to medium and process the melon and ginger.
	6 Stir in the mint, pour into 2 glasses, and enjoy!

Per serving: Calories 183 (From Fat 10); Fat 1g (Saturated 0g); Cholesterol 0mg; Sodium 19mg; Carbohydrate 45g (Dietary Fiber 4g); Protein 4g.

Tip: If you prefer, use a whole sprig of fresh mint and juice it with the melon so that the texture of the chopped mint isn't rough in the drink.

Opt for organic

The word *organic* is meant to define a set of standards for the methods, practices, and substances that are used to grow and process agricultural products. Essentially, it means that ethical, sustainable practices are used in farming. It also means that consumers can be confident that none of the following will be used on fruit and vegetables:

✔ Chemical pesticides and fertilizers

✔ Sewage sludge

✔ Synthetic hormones

✔ Genetically engineered plants

✔ Cloned animals

✔ Excessive food processing, artificial ingredients, preservatives, or irradiation

✔ Antibiotics to prevent disease

Focusing on Digestive Fruit Juices

As one of the key body systems, the digestive tract is important because it breaks down the food that you eat and gets the nutrients into the bloodstream, where they're distributed to the cells that require and use them. On a basic level, you can feel bloated or even experience unpleasant pain or gas when your digestive system isn't working at its optimum.

Enzymes in some fruits, bacteria in yogurt, and the stimulating actions of some herbs assist the body in its daily job of digesting the food you eat.

Eat fruits separately: Food combining 101

If you've experienced digestive problems (such as bloating, gas, cramps, diarrhea, and indigestion), or if you begin to experience them after juicing, your problem may lie in *when* you're eating certain types of foods, not *what* you're eating, especially if your diet consists of whole grains, fruits, vegetables, legumes, nuts, seeds, herbs, and not a lot of refined foods.

Sudden drinking of pure raw fruit and/or vegetable juices can cause the body to have problems where none existed before. This is due to the concentration of the enzymes in juices and the absence of fiber and cellulose, which mitigate some of their effects.

Food combining involves eating different types of food in a specific order so that the various digestive enzymes for each type of food are released when that food is in the gut. Food combining has been credited with relieving fatigue, food allergies, and, in some cases, inflammatory bowel and peptic ulcer, in addition to digestive problems.

Food combining is a complex topic, so I'm only going to touch on the issues most relevant to juicing, which are about fruits:

Eat fruits separately. The acids in fruit prevent carbohydrate and protein digestion because the enzyme *ptyalin,* which breaks down carbohydrates and protein, requires an alkaline medium and fruit is acid. This means that whenever carbohydrate and protein foods are eaten with fruit, they won't be digested, so they'll sit and putrefy either in the stomach or the intestines. And if that's not bad enough, fruit takes the least time to be digested; if it sits on top of slower digesting fats, protein, and carbohydrate foods in the gut, it will start to ferment those foods.

Bottom line: If you experience digestive problems, try eating fruit or drinking fruit juice at least 30 minutes to 1 hour *before* or at least 2 hours *after* a meal, and keep fruits separate from vegetables in the same drink.

If you want to investigate the fascinating topic of food combining, check out *The Complete Book of Food Combining,* by Kathryn Marsden (Piatkus Books).

Papaya Pride

Prep time: About 2 min • **Juicing time:** 2 min • **Yield:** 2 servings

Ingredients	Directions
2 papayas 2 mangos 1 lime ½ pineapple	*1* Peel the papayas and mangos and remove the pits.
	2 Peel the lime, leaving the white pith on.
	3 Cut the pineapple flesh into wedges to fit the juicer feed tube.
	4 Turn on the juicer and place a jug under the spout.
	5 Working on a slow speed, process the papayas, mangos, and lime.
	6 Increase the speed to medium and process the pineapple.
	7 Stir the drink, pour into 2 glasses, and enjoy!

Per serving: Calories 321 (From Fat 13); Fat 1g (Saturated 0g); Cholesterol 0mg; Sodium 14mg; Carbohydrate 83g (Dietary Fiber 4g); Protein 3g.

Tip: To trim pineapple, cut the top and the base off the pineapple and cut the pineapple in half lengthwise. Wrap one half and set aside in the refrigerator. Stand the other pineapple half up and cut away and discard the outer skin.

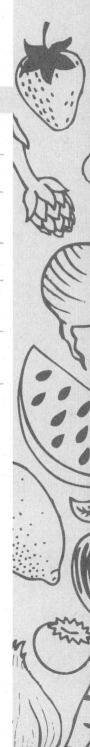

Peppermint Kiwi

Prep time: About 3 min • **Juicing time:** 2 min • **Yield:** 2 servings

Ingredients	Directions
3 kiwifruits	*1* Peel the kiwifruits and papayas.
1 sprig fresh peppermint	
2 papayas	*2* Peel the lime, leaving the white pith on.
1 lime	
¼ pineapple	*3* Cut the top and the base off the pineapple and cut the pineapple in half lengthwise. Cut each half in half lengthwise. Wrap 3 quarters and set aside in the refrigerator. Stand up the remaining pineapple quarter and cut away the outer skin; discard.
½ cup sparkling mineral water	
	4 Turn on the juicer and place a jug under the spout.
	5 Working on a slow speed, process the kiwifruits, peppermint, papayas, and lime.
	6 Increase the speed to medium and process the pineapple.
	7 Stir in the mineral water, pour into 2 glasses, and enjoy!

Per serving: Calories 243 (From Fat 12); Fat 1g (Saturated 0g); Cholesterol 0mg; Sodium 11mg; Carbohydrate 63g (Dietary Fiber 4g); Protein 2g.

Tip: Sip on this drink up to one hour before eating and it will aid your digestion.

Vary It: If you don't have access to fresh peppermint, use up to ¼ teaspoon dried peppermint in this refreshing beverage.

Trying Some Immune-Boosting Juices

Your immune system includes your body's skin covering, nose, mouth and throat tissue, lymph nodes, and organs including your spleen and tonsils. This complex defense system holds the key to resisting infections, allergies, and chronic illness. It protects against and attacks viruses, bacteria, parasites, and fungi, enabling your body to resist all invading microorganisms.

One of the first ways to support your immune system is to wash: Wash your hands frequently, wash fresh produce (peel if non-organic), and keep your kitchen and utensils spotlessly clean. The next step is to add plenty of colorful fruits, especially berries, and vegetables to your diet and then boost the effectiveness of those naturally protective foods with flu- and disease-fighting ingredients.

You can immune-boost any fresh juice by adding one or two of the following ingredients:

- ¼ to ½ cup probiotic yogurt or kefir containing *Lactobacillus reuteri*
- ¼ to ½ clove fresh garlic, minced
- A handful of fresh kale or Swiss chard leaves (including stalks)
- A ½ cup freshly brewed (chilled) black or green tea
- 20 drops Echinacea
- ¼ teaspoon ground cinnamon or minced green herb (such as oregano, sage, and thyme)

Refer to Chapter 21 for more tips on how to boost your immunity.

Radiant Rainbow

Prep time: About 3 min • **Juicing time:** 2 min • **Yield:** 2 servings

Ingredients	Directions
½ **lemon**	*1* Peel the lemon, leaving on the white pith.
½ **cucumber**	
3 mature kale leaves, stems intact	*2* Peel the cucumber.
2 pears	*3* Turn on the juicer and place a jug under the spout.
1 apple	*4* Working on a slow speed, process the lemon, cucumber, and kale.
3 carrots	
1 small beet	*5* Increase the speed to medium and process the pears and apple.
1 piece (1-inch) peeled fresh ginger	
	6 Increase the speed to high and process the carrots, beet, and ginger.
	7 Stir the drink, pour into 2 glasses, and enjoy!

Per serving: Calories 230 (From Fat 10); Fat 1g (Saturated 0g); Cholesterol 0mg; Sodium 112mg; Carbohydrate 58g (Dietary Fiber 12g); Protein 5g.

Tip: Using baby kale in this recipe makes the overall taste less assertive. If you use the smaller, more tender baby kale leaves, double or triple the amount called for in this recipe.

Berry Beetilicious

Prep time: About 3 min • **Juicing time:** 2 min • **Yield:** 2 servings

Ingredients	Directions
1 orange	*1* Peel the orange and lemon, leaving the white pith on.
½ lemon	
1 apple	*2* Peel the apple (if not organic), cut into quarters, and remove the core and seeds.
1 cup mixed berries, fresh or frozen, thawed	
1 piece (1-inch) peeled fresh ginger	*3* Turn on the juicer and place a jug under the spout.
3 carrots	*4* Working on a slow speed, process the berries, orange, and lemon.
1 medium beet	
	5 Increase the speed to medium and process the apple and ginger.
	6 Increase the speed to high and process the carrots and beet.
	7 Stir the drink, pour into 2 glasses, and enjoy!

Per serving: Calories 186 (From Fat 8); Fat 1g (Saturated 0g); Cholesterol 0mg; Sodium 98mg; Carbohydrate 47g (Dietary Fiber 2g); Protein 3g.

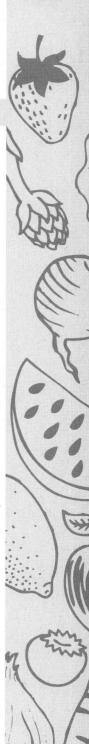

Making Some Fruit Mocktails, Cocktail Mixers, and Punches

They taste delicious. They won't give you a hangover or make you prance around with a lampshade on your head. They feed your cells and nourish your body in miraculous ways. You can drink them and drive home. What's not to like about mocktails?

Using fresh fruit juices as the mixer in alcoholic drinks is smart. The vitamins — especially the antioxidant vitamin A — help to soothe nerves and replenish vital nutrients and water that alcohol depletes. You get natural sugars instead of empty calories in sodas. And they taste so darned good!

The punch bowl is festive and it can be the center of a lively party. Offering a nonalcoholic punch is a responsible host's job, and designated drivers will be thankful that you made it with fresh, refreshing ingredients.

Creating a health hub

For success in juicing and to stay motivated and firmly develop the juicing habit, you need to get up close and personal with your juicer. The first rule of juicing is that the juicer takes center stage on the kitchen counter and is in full view all the time. When you accept that the juicing machine will always be there, reminding you of its noble cause, you can think carefully about how you work and what will streamline the process of juicing.

Run through the juicing process and organize your juicing equipment so that you work clean and uncluttered. Keep a peeling knife and a larger vegetable knife sharpened and at hand at the juicing center or what I like to think of as the health hub. You need a large cutting board and a long-handled brush, as well as a jug to collect the juice if your juicer doesn't come with its own jug. A compost bucket and a supply of plastic bags for collecting and saving the pulp are essential (see Chapter 13). Situate the juicer as close to the sink and to your glasses as you can (you may have to rearrange some cupboards). This will save time when it comes to serving the juice and cleaning up.

If you can, position the juicer on the counter between the sink and the refrigerator because most of the fresh fruit and vegetables will need to be chilled. Reserve a shelf in your refrigerator, preferably at eye level, for juicing ingredients. The more prominent the ingredients are, the more likely you'll be to use them.

Piña-Strawberry Colada

Prep time: About 3 min • **Juicing time:** 2 min • **Yield:** 3 servings

Ingredients	Directions
4 cups strawberries	**1** Wash the strawberries under gently streaming water, hull, and pat dry.
½ lemon	
½ pineapple	**2** Peel the lemon, leaving the white pith on.
½ cup coconut cream	**3** Cut the top and the base off the pineapple and cut the pineapple in half lengthwise. Wrap one half and set aside in the refrigerator. Stand up the other half and cut away and discard the outer skin. Cut the pineapple flesh into wedges to fit the juicer feed tube.
	4 Turn on the juicer and place a jug under the spout.
	5 Working on a slow speed, process the strawberries and lemon.
	6 Increase the speed to medium and process the pineapple.
	7 Stir in coconut cream, pour into 2 glasses, and enjoy!

Per serving: Calories 197 (From Fat 89); Fat 10g (Saturated 8g); Cholesterol 0mg; Sodium 28mg; Carbohydrate 29g (Dietary Fiber 2g); Protein 3g.

Tip: Coconut cream is found in the same section of the supermarket as coconut milk. It's made in exactly the same way as coconut milk, but with less water, which makes it thicker in drinks. Use coconut milk if you can't find coconut cream.

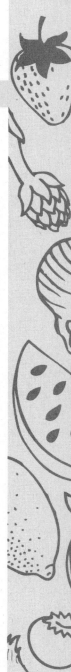

Skoal!

Prep time: About 3 min • **Juicing time:** 2 min • **Yield:** 2 servings

Ingredients	Directions
2 oranges	**1** Peel the oranges and grapefruit, leaving the white pith on.
1 ruby grapefruit	
1 mango	**2** Peel the mango and remove the pit.
1 cup sparkling grape juice or mineral water	**3** Turn on the juicer and place a jug under the spout.
	4 Working on a slow speed, process the oranges and grapefruit.
	5 Increase the speed to medium and process the mango.
	6 Stir in the grape juice, pour into 2 glasses, and enjoy!

Per serving: Calories 170 (From Fat 5); Fat 1g (Saturated 0g); Cholesterol 0mg; Sodium 2mg; Carbohydrate 44g (Dietary Fiber 4g); Protein 5g.

Red Zinger Mixer

Prep time: About 4 min • **Juicing time:** 2 min • **Yield:** 2 servings

Ingredients	Directions
2 pomegranates 2 oranges 1 cup raspberries 2 ounces vodka, rum, or gin	**1** Break apart each of the pomegranates into 4 pieces and pull out the red seeds. Discard the rind and the white membrane.
	2 Peel the oranges, leaving the white pith on.
	3 Wash the raspberries under gently streaming water; pat dry.
	4 Turn on the juicer and place a jug under the spout.
	5 Working on a slow speed, process the oranges and raspberries.
	6 Increase the speed to medium and process the pomegranate seeds.
	7 Stir in the alcohol, pour into 2 glasses, and enjoy!

Per serving: Calories 262 (From Fat 9); Fat 1g (Saturated 0g); Cholesterol 0mg; Sodium 5mg; Carbohydrate 49g (Dietary Fiber 3g); Protein 4g.

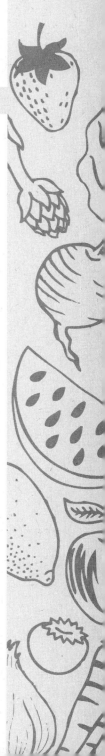

Gingered Orange Mixer

Prep time: About 2 min • **Juicing time:** 2 min • **Yield:** 2 servings

Ingredients	Directions
2 oranges	*1* Peel the oranges, leaving the white pith on.
2 red plums	
1 piece (1-inch) peeled fresh ginger	*2* Cut the plums in half and remove the stone.
3 pears	*3* Cut the pears if necessary to fit the juicer feed tube.
2 ounces vodka, rum, or gin	*4* Turn on the juicer and place a jug under the spout.
	5 Working on a slow speed, process the oranges.
	6 Increase the speed to medium and process the plums, ginger, and pears.
	7 Stir in the alcohol, pour into 2 glasses, and enjoy!

Per serving: Calories 313 (From Fat 14); Fat 2g (Saturated 0g); Cholesterol 0mg; Sodium 1mg; Carbohydrate 62g (Dietary Fiber 4g); Protein 3g.

Cool Watermelon Punch

Prep time: About 6 min • **Juicing time:** 2 min • **Yield:** 6 servings

Ingredients	Directions
1 watermelon	*1* Cut the watermelon in half lengthwise. Trim away the top and bottom. Cut each half in half lengthwise. Trim away the rind and any white flesh; discard. Cut into wedges to fit the feed tube of the juicer.
3 red grapefruits	
3 oranges	
2 papayas	*2* Peel the grapefruits, oranges, and lime, leaving the white pith on.
1 lime	
4 cups ice cubes	*3* Peel the papayas.
	4 Turn on the juicer and place a jug under the spout.
	5 Working on a slow speed, process the watermelon, grapefruits, oranges, papayas, and lime.
	6 Pour the punch into a container with a tight-fitting lid and refrigerate until guests arrive.
	7 When ready to serve, shake or stir the punch and pour into a punch bowl. Add ice and enjoy!

Per serving: Calories 333 (From Fat 2); Fat 0g (Saturated 0g); Cholesterol 0mg; Sodium 18mg; Carbohydrate 83g (Dietary Fiber 4g); Protein 6g.

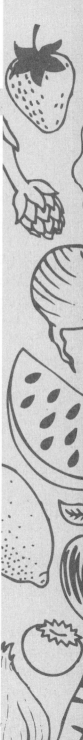

Apple Melon Fizz Punch

Prep time: About 6 min • **Juicing time:** 2 min • **Yield:** 6 servings

Ingredients	Directions
1 honeydew, musk, or cantaloupe melon	*1* Cut the melon in half, scoop out the seeds and trim away the rind; discard. Cut the melon flesh into wedges to fit the juicer feed tube.
2 oranges	
6 apples	*2* Peel the oranges, leaving the white pith on.
1 piece (2-inches) peeled fresh ginger	*3* Cut the apples to fit the juicer feed tube.
2 cups carbonated water	*4* Turn on the juicer and place a jug under the spout.
4 cups ice cubes	*5* Working on a slow speed, process the melon and oranges.
	6 Pour the punch into a container with a tight-fitting lid and refrigerate until guests arrive.
	7 When ready to serve, shake or stir the punch and pour into a punch bowl. Stir in carbonated water, add ice, and enjoy!

Per serving: Calories 178 (From Fat 7); Fat 1g (Saturated 0g); Cholesterol 0mg; Sodium 22mg; Carbohydrate 46g (Dietary Fiber 2g); Protein 2g.

Tip: You may find that adding apple in a juice produces a bit of foam. Simply give the juice a quick stir with a whisk before pouring into glasses.

Using natural digestive ingredients

If you suffer with a weak digestive system, some natural foods can help with the problem. For most people, a lack of fiber is one of the key causes of poor digestion, so increase your consumption of beans, whole grains, and fresh fruits and vegetables. You'll see a difference almost immediately. A healthy digestive tract prevents diverticulosis and colon cancer, two totally preventable digestive diseases.

Here are some fruits, vegetables, and herbs that will increase your digestive function. Juice them or use them in smoothies:

✔ **Kiwifruits:** Eating kiwifruits will help cleanse the system and aid digestion. Rich in vitamin C and the antioxidant vitamin E, they also are high in potassium and contain calcium and dietary fiber.

✔ **Papayas:** The enzyme papain from papayas is used in digestive remedies. High in vitamins A and C, papayas are an excellent addition to juice ingredients.

✔ **Pineapples:** Bromelain is the anti-inflammatory enzyme found in pineapples that is so helpful in digestion. Pineapples also are a good source of vitamin C.

✔ **Fennel:** Juice from the bulb has a gentle action on digestion, but the ground seeds will soothe discomfort from heartburn and indigestion. For after-dinner relief, stir up to ½ teaspoon ground fennel seeds into a juice or smoothie.

✔ **Calendula:** Aids digestion by stimulating bile production. Stir up to ½ teaspoon dried calendula petals into a juice or smoothie.

✔ **Cinnamon:** Use dried ground cinnamon in juices or smoothies as a gentle aid to digestion. Stir ¼ teaspoon into drinks and use as aperitif or after-dinner digestive.

✔ **Dandelion root:** Use as a natural laxative and to stimulate the liver and gall bladder to produce more bile. It also helps reduce high blood pressure. Purchase ground, dried dandelion root, and stir up to ½ teaspoon into drinks.

✔ **German chamomile:** German chamomile soothes stomach pain caused by inflammation or gas. It's taken as a tea, or the tea may be used as the liquid in a soothing smoothie.

✔ **Ginger:** An excellent addition to juices or smoothies because it stimulates blood flow to the digestive system and increases absorption of nutrients. Use it for indigestion and to assist in the breakdown of fatty foods. Juice the fresh peeled root or stir ¼ teaspoon ground, dried ginger into drinks.

✔ **Licorice:** Soothes stomach ulcers and indigestion but should be avoided if you have high blood pressure. Stir ¼ teaspoon ground, dried licorice into drinks.

✔ **Peppermint:** Increases the flow of bile by stimulating the liver and gallbladder. Juice fresh peppermint or stir 1 to 3 teaspoons chopped fresh peppermint into after-dinner drinks.

✔ **Turmeric:** Used as a digestive aid because it stimulates the liver and gallbladder. Stir up to ¼ teaspoon ground, dried turmeric into drinks.

Chapter 13

Blending Some Vegetable Juices

*V*egetables are packed with antioxidants, anti-inflammatory, and anti-cancer components, along with other high-powered nutrients that keep your body fit. Just like fruit, you need five or six servings of fresh vegetables every day, and juices are a tasty and easy way to ensure that your daily quota is met. Vegetable juices are great at breakfast, but they can supplement or substitute for a quick and nutritious lunch or light dinner. Fit them into your life and feel the energy and vitality they bring! I provide a plethora of vegetable juices in this chapter to help you start.

So, how do vegetables differ from fruit? Because of their low acidity, vegetable juices offer a rainbow of goodness that you can consume any time of the day, with meals or as snacks, all day long.

Proteins and fat take the longest time to be digested and move out of the stomach, but fruit is digested very quickly. For this reason, it may be best if you first consume fruit in the morning after rising or an hour or two before or after meals. If you eat fruit too close to a meal, the fruit tends to sit on top of food in the gut, causing it to putrefy and form gas.

Waking Up with Breakfast Juices

Studies have proven that eating low-starch, high-protein breakfasts increases alertness and energy in the morning — and the positive effect actually stays with you and keeps you from craving high-calorie snacks in the afternoon and into the early evening! So, I include a protein in each of these breakfast juices so that you can start your day with a high-protein beverage and enjoy a slimmer body, and at the same time, a more energetic life.

In the morning, combining vegetables with some fruit can help to acclimate your taste buds to the savory side of vegetables. If your buds are already vegetable friendly, you can cut down or eliminate the fruit in these recipes, but you may like to keep them along with the hit of fructose they bring.

Sunriser

Prep time: About 3 min • **Juicing time:** 2 min • **Yield:** 2 servings

Ingredients	Directions
2 oranges	*1* Peel the oranges and lemon, leaving the white pith on.
½ lemon	
½ red pepper, stem removed	*2* Cut the red pepper to fit the juicer feed tube.
4 carrots	*3* Turn on the juicer and place a jug under the spout.
2 celery stalks	
1 piece (1-inch) peeled ginger	*4* Working on a slow speed, process the oranges, lemon, and red pepper.
¼ cup soy or whey protein powder	*5* Increase the speed to medium and process the carrots, celery, and ginger.
	6 Stir the protein powder into the drink, pour into 2 glasses, and enjoy!

Per serving: *Calories 211 (From Fat 11); Fat 1g (Saturated 0g); Cholesterol 0mg; Sodium 223mg; Carbohydrate 39g (Dietary Fiber 4g); Protein 14g.*

Tip: Use whey or soy protein powder in any of the recipes in this chapter, but if you can, purchase an organic soy protein powder because non-organic soybeans are genetically modified and often are grown with a lot of herbicides.

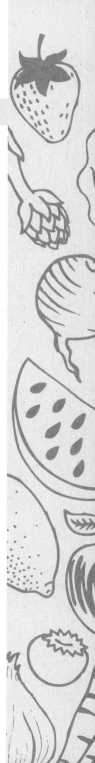

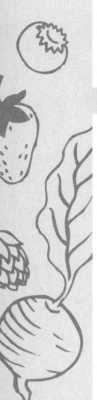

Beet in Motion

Prep time: About 3 min • **Juicing time:** 2 min • **Yield:** 2 servings

Ingredients	Directions
1 lime	**1** Peel the lime, leaving the white pith on.
3 carrots	**2** Scrub the beets and cut them if necessary to fit the juicer feed tube.
2 celery stalks	
2 apples	**3** Cut the apples if necessary to fit the juicer feed tube.
2 beets	
¼ cup soft tofu	**4** Turn on the juicer and place a jug under the spout.
	5 Working on a slow speed, process the lime.
	6 Increase the speed to medium and process the carrots, celery, and apples.
	7 Increase the speed to high and process the beets.
	8 Using a fork, stir the tofu into the drink. Pour into 2 glasses and enjoy!

Per serving: Calories 192 (From Fat 15); Fat 2g (Saturated 0g); Cholesterol 0mg; Sodium 153mg; Carbohydrate 45g (Dietary Fiber 4g); Protein 4g.

Warning: Take it easy with beets. Raw beets have a laxative effect on your digestive system, so try one or even one-half beet in this recipe until your body adjusts.

Tip: If you find that the tofu is too lumpy, pour the juice and the tofu into a blender and process to combine into a smooth and drinkable beverage.

Tip: If you have beets with the green leaves attached, keep them on and juice them with the beets.

Brassy Brassica

Prep time: About 2 min • **Juicing time:** 2 min • **Yield:** 2 servings

Ingredients	Directions
½ **lemon**	*1* Peel the lemon, leaving the white pith on.
4 **broccoli spears**	
¼ **green cabbage**	*2* Cut the broccoli, cabbage, and apples, if necessary to fit the juicer feed tube.
2 **apples**	
2 **carrots**	*3* Turn on the juicer and place a jug under the spout.
¼ **cup finely ground almonds**	
	4 Working on a slow speed, process the lemon.
	5 Increase the speed to medium and process the broccoli, cabbage, apples, and carrots.
	6 Stir the almonds into the drink, pour into 2 glasses, and enjoy!

Per serving: Calories 443 (From Fat 128); Fat 14g (Saturated 1g); Cholesterol 0mg; Sodium 112mg; Carbohydrate 79g (Dietary Fiber 10g); Protein 13g.

Tip: Use any of the Brassica plants — broccoli, cauliflower, cabbage, kale, turnip, or Brussels sprouts — in this drink. The apples and carrots sweeten the drink naturally, but for sensitive palates, add a teaspoon of honey.

Note: Using cruciferous vegetables like broccoli, cabbage, Brussels sprouts, and cauliflower will make a slightly sulfurous and, therefore, stinky juice, but this is the active healing ingredients at work.

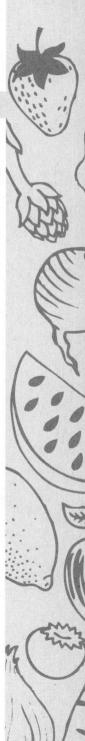

Gingered Greens

Prep time: About 3 min • **Juicing time:** 2 min • **Yield:** 2 servings

Ingredients	Directions
2 cups packed spinach	*1* Wash the spinach and kale under gently streaming water; pat dry.
2 kale or Swiss chard leaves	
½ English cucumber	*2* Peel the lime, leaving the white pith on.
½ lime	
2 broccoli spears	*3* Cut the broccoli and apples, if necessary, to fit the juicer feed tube.
1 piece (1-inch) peeled fresh ginger	
2 apples	*4* Turn on the juicer and place a jug under the spout.
¼ cup cottage or ricotta cheese	
	5 Working on a slow speed, process the spinach, kale, cucumber, and lime.
	6 Increase the speed to medium and process the broccoli, ginger, and apples.
	7 Using a fork, stir the cheese into the drink. Pour into 2 glasses and enjoy!

Per serving: Calories 144 (From Fat 13); Fat 1g (Saturated 1g); Cholesterol 2mg; Sodium 249mg; Carbohydrate 30g (Dietary Fiber 3g); Protein 7g.

Tip: English cucumbers are mild, seedless, and, best of all, skinny, so they easily fit most juicer feed tubes. You can use regular garden cucumbers, but you'll need to remove most of the bitter peel and cut them to fit the juicer feed tube.

Tip: If you find that the cottage or ricotta cheese is too lumpy, pour the juice and the cheese into a blender and process to combine into a smooth and drinkable beverage.

Adding Vegetables to Your Diet with Lunch and Dinner Juices

On the go? Too busy/hot/lazy to cook? Don't want to grab a high-carb, high-calorie sandwich or burger? Need a shot of energy? Why not try drinking your lunch or dinner instead?

I include a small amount of protein in these drinks because it takes longer to digest and, therefore, stays with you until your next snack or meal.

Slip grasses and herbs between celery or apple

If you've ever tried to juice cabbage or lettuce leaves, green grasses, or herbs, you likely found that they jammed in the basket and just made a mess. Usually, cabbage is cut into wedges and it passes through the juicing basket easily, but if you don't want to add too much strong cabbage taste to a juice and you have a few large outer leaves that you want to combine with other ingredients in a juice, the best way to get the most out of the leaves is to roll them into a tight, long, cylindrical shape and guide them through the feed tube using celery stalks, carrots, or apple wedges.

Herb sprigs and cereal grasses are more delicate, so they're more difficult to juice without the benefit of a special attachment. I've found that if I wedge a handful of green grasses or herbs in the natural groove of a celery stalk, the celery keeps the grass in place long enough for the juice to be extracted.

There is another way to "juice" wheatgrass and herbs using a blender. This method is more efficient in extracting the essential and active elements in wheatgrass. Here's how to do it:

1. **In the blender container, combine 1½ cups water with 2 to 3 cups fresh wheatgrass.**

2. **Process the mixture on high for 30 to 40 seconds or until the grass is liquefied.**

3. **Line a sieve with a layer of cheesecloth and set it over a large bowl.**

4. **Pour the wheatgrass and water through the sieve into the bowl.**

5. **Squeeze the cheesecloth to remove all the moisture from the wheatgrass.**

6. **Blend ¼ to ½ of the wheatgrass juice into fresh fruit or vegetable juice or use as part of the liquid in smoothies.**

Waldorf Salad

Prep time: About 2 min • **Juicing time:** 2 min • **Yield:** 2 servings

Ingredients	Directions
½ head green cabbage	**1** Cut the cabbage and apples if necessary to fit the juicer feed tube.
3 carrots	
2 apples	**2** Turn on the juicer and place a jug under the spout.
½ cup plain low-fat yogurt	
¼ teaspoon ground fennel seeds	**3** Working on medium speed, process the cabbage, carrots, and apples.
2 tablespoons finely ground walnuts	**4** Stir yogurt and fennel seeds into the drink and pour into 2 glasses. Garnish each glass with 1 tablespoon of chopped walnuts and enjoy!

Per serving: Calories 250 (From Fat 50); Fat 6g (Saturated 1g); Cholesterol 4mg; Sodium 116mg; Carbohydrate 48g (Dietary Fiber 6g); Protein 9g.

Sesame Says Me

Prep time: About 2 min • **Juicing time:** 2 min • **Yield:** 2 servings

Ingredients	Directions
1 handful fresh green beans	**1** Cut the apple, if necessary to fit the juicer feed tube.
1 cup Brussels sprouts	
6 carrots	**2** Turn on the juicer and place a jug under the spout.
1 apple	**3** Working on a medium speed, process the beans and Brussels sprouts, using the carrots and apple to push them through the feed tube.
1 tablespoon Tahini	
1 tablespoon plain or toasted sesame seeds	**4** Whisk the Tahini into the drink and pour into 2 glasses. Garnish each glass with sesame seeds and enjoy!

Per serving: Calories 226 (From Fat 63); Fat 7g (Saturated 1g); Cholesterol 0mg; Sodium 82mg; Carbohydrate 40g (Dietary Fiber 5g); Protein 7g.

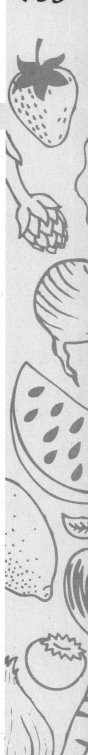

Winter Roots

Prep time: About 3 min • **Juicing time:** 2 min • **Yield:** 2 servings

Ingredients	Directions
¼ fennel bulb, stems and leaves intact	*1* Leave the stems and fernlike leaves on the fennel bulb for juicing. Cut the bulb in half and cut one-half in half again. Wrap one-half and one-quarter and set aside in the refrigerator.
3 carrots	
2 apples	
2 parsnips	*2* Cut the remaining quarter fennel and apples if necessary, to fit the juicer feed tube.
1 cup rutabaga or turnip cubes	
¼ cup cottage or ricotta cheese	*3* Turn on the juicer and place a jug under the spout.
	4 Working on a medium speed, process the fennel, carrots, apples, and parsnips.
	5 Increase the speed to high and process the rutabaga.
	6 Using a fork, stir the cheese into the drink. Pour into 2 glasses and enjoy!

Per serving: Calories 304 (From Fat 17); Fat 2g (Saturated 1g); Cholesterol 2mg; Sodium 182mg; Carbohydrate 69g (Dietary Fiber 7g); Protein 8g.

Tip: If you find that the cottage or ricotta cheese is too lumpy, pour the juice and the cheese into a blender and process to combine into a smooth and drinkable beverage.

Smokin' Peppers

Prep time: About 3 min • **Juicing time:** 2 min • **Yield:** 2 servings

Ingredients	Directions
1 medium tomato	**1** Cut the tomato, peppers, zucchini, and cucumber if necessary to fit the juicer feed tube.
3 red bell peppers, jalapeño peppers, or habanero chile peppers	
2 zucchini	**2** Scoop out the seeds and trim away the rind from the melon. Discard the seeds and rind. Cut the melon flesh into wedges to fit the juicer feed tube.
1 small to medium cucumber	
½ muskmelon1 clove garlic	**3** Turn on the juicer and place a jug under the spout.
¼ cup crumbled feta cheese	**4** Working on a slow speed, process the tomato, peppers, zucchini, and cucumber.
1 tablespoon chopped fresh cilantro	
	5 Increase the speed to medium and process the melon and garlic.
	6 Using a fork, stir the cheese into the drink. Pour into 2 glasses, garnish each with cilantro, and enjoy!

Per serving: Calories 201 (From Fat 48); Fat 5g (Saturated 3g); Cholesterol 17mg; Sodium 240mg; Carbohydrate 35g (Dietary Fiber 3g); Protein 9g.

Tip: If you find that the feta cheese is too lumpy, pour the juice and the cheese into a blender and process to combine into a smooth and drinkable beverage.

Vary It: You can make this drink smokin' hot or sweetly tame simply by varying the type of pepper you use. Red bell peppers are sweet, jalapeño peppers add a bit of heat, and habanero chile peppers are three-alarm hot.

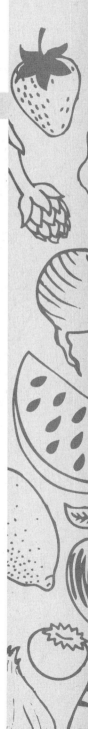

Healthy Giant

Prep time: About 3 min • **Juicing time:** 2 min • **Yield:** 2 servings

Ingredients	Directions
2 medium tomatoes	*1* Cut the tomatoes and broccoli if necessary to fit the juicer feed tube.
1 cup packed spinach	
3 broccoli spears	*2* Turn on the juicer and place a jug under the spout.
2 celery stalks	
1 piece (1-inch) peeled ginger	*3* Working on a slow speed, process the tomato, spinach, broccoli, celery, ginger, and zucchini.
1 zucchini	
¼ cup plain yogurt	*4* Whisk in the yogurt. Pour the drink into 2 glasses, garnish each with parsley, and enjoy!
1 tablespoon finely chopped fresh parsley	

Per serving: Calories 91 (From Fat 13); Fat 1g (Saturated 1g); Cholesterol 2mg; Sodium 116mg; Carbohydrate 17g (Dietary Fiber 1g); Protein 6g.

Balancing sweet fruits with lemon and vegetables

You'll likely progress from exclusively juicing fruit to juicing some vegetables with fruit to mostly juicing vegetables. This progression is important because fruit is higher in sugar than vegetables, and vegetables help balance your body's pH, making them the preferred juice. Early on, you should set and work toward the goal of juicing vegetables to fruit in a two-to-one ratio. You can get there by using two vegetables and one fruit in a single drink or by consuming two vegetable juices for every fruit juice in a day.

Fruits and fruit juices have definite advantages (their antioxidants for one). But fruit juices, because they're made from several whole fruits and because they aren't bound up in the complex carbohydrates and fiber of the whole fruit, are higher in sugars than vegetable juices, so they tend to spike blood sugar levels and increase insulin levels.

One way to help you move toward a love of vegetable juice is to include lemon with all juices, especially those that are exclusively fruit. Start by including a quarter lemon with the white pith intact with fruit ingredients. When you become accustomed to that amount, you can increase to one-half lemon with the white pith intact. Surprisingly, the taste isn't pucker-tart. Instead, the lemon simply balances the cloyingly sweet flavor of all-fruit juices.

Creamy Beet

Prep time: About 3 min • **Juicing time:** 2 min • **Yield:** 2 servings

Ingredients	Directions
1 cup packed spinach	*1* Peel the lemon, leaving the white pith on.
½ lemon	
4 green onions	*2* Cut the zucchini and beets if necessary to fit the juicer feed tube.
2 celery stalks	
1 zucchini	*3* Turn on the juicer and place a jug under the spout.
3 beets	
1 cup plain yogurt	*4* Working on a slow speed, process the spinach, lemon, onions, celery, and zucchini. Use the celery and zucchini to help push the spinach through the feed tube.
1 tablespoon chopped fresh basil	
	5 Increase the speed to high and process the beets.
	6 Whisk in the yogurt. Pour the drink into 2 glasses, garnish each with basil, and enjoy!

Per serving: Calories 188 (From Fat 23); Fat 3g (Saturated 1g); Cholesterol 7mg; Sodium 317mg; Carbohydrate 33g (Dietary Fiber 2g); Protein 12g.

Tip: Alternate the spinach with the onions and celery to get the most juice from the leaves.

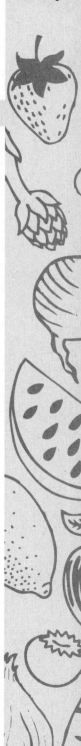

Blending Some Snack Juices

You get energy from the foods that you eat. The same basic rule of computers applies to your body: Garbage in, garbage out.

Juicing is a great way to quickly send nutrients to cells via the bloodstream, without taxing the digestive system. Drinking juices for between-meal snacks quickly brings your energy levels back to optimum. And it gets better, because by gradually releasing blood sugars into your body, the effect lasts longer than it would if you were to eat a refined-sugar snack.

Plus, pure vegetable juices don't add a caloric burden to your daily food intake. You can drink them morning, afternoon, and night without adding excessive amounts of fat or sugar to your system.

The following recipes offer you an assortment of vegetable-based juices that you can drink for snacks, either midmorning or midday, and give your body the nutrients that it needs.

Seed Power

Prep time: About 2 min • **Juicing time:** 2 min • **Yield:** 2 servings

Ingredients	Directions
2 kale or Swiss chard leaves	*1* Cut the broccoli and apple if necessary, to fit the juicer feed tube.
½ English cucumber	
4 carrots	*2* Roll each kale leaf lengthwise along the stem to make it easier to juice.
3 broccoli spears	
1 apple	*3* Turn on the juicer and place a jug under the spout.
¼ cup finely ground raw almonds	*4* Working on a slow speed, process the kale leaves, using the cucumber to push them through the feed tube.
2 teaspoons raw pumpkin seeds	
2 teaspoons raw sunflower seeds	*5* Increase the speed to medium and process the carrots, broccoli, and apple.
	6 Stir the almonds into the drink. Pour into 2 glasses, garnish each with pumpkin and sunflower seeds, and enjoy!

Per serving: Calories 227 (From Fat 86); Fat 10g (Saturated 1g); Cholesterol 0mg; Sodium 69mg; Carbohydrate 33g (Dietary Fiber 3g); Protein 8g.

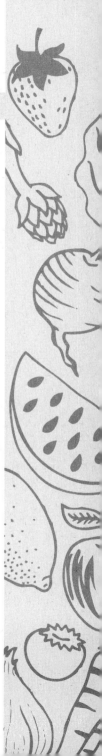

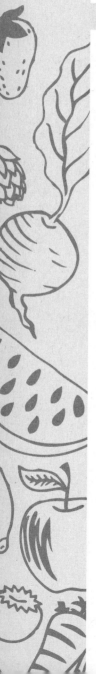

Veggie Power

Prep time: About 2 min • **Juicing time:** 2 min • **Yield:** 2 servings

Ingredients	Directions
½ **lemon**	**1** Peel the lemon, leaving the white pith on.
½ **small red cabbage**	
2 **pears**	**2** Cut the cabbage and pears if necessary, to fit the juicer feed tube.
2 **carrots**	
2 **celery stalks**	**3** Turn on the juicer and place a jug under the spout.
2 **teaspoons raw sunflower seeds**	**4** Working on a slow speed, process the lemon.
	5 Increase the speed to medium and process the cabbage, pears, carrots, and celery.
	6 Stir the drink, pour into 2 glasses, garnish each with sunflower seeds, and enjoy!

Per serving: Calories 192 (From Fat 23); Fat 3g (Saturated 0g); Cholesterol 0mg; Sodium 94mg; Carbohydrate 44g (Dietary Fiber 4g); Protein 4g.

Calcium Rules

Prep time: About 2 min • **Juicing time:** 2 min • **Yield:** 2 servings

Ingredients	Directions
4 broccoli spears 1 small bok choy	*1* Cut the broccoli, bok choy, and pears if necessary, to fit the juicer feed tube.
3 celery stalks 3 pears	*2* Turn on the juicer and place a jug under the spout.
2 tablespoons finely ground almonds	*3* Working on a medium speed, process the broccoli, bok choy, celery, and pears.
1 tablespoon finely crumbled feta cheese	*4* Stir the almonds into the drink. Pour into 2 glasses, garnish each with feta cheese, and enjoy!

Per serving: Calories 283 (From Fat 56); Fat 6g (Saturated 1g); Cholesterol 4mg; Sodium 428mg; Carbohydrate 55g (Dietary Fiber 4g); Protein 12g.

Tip: Adults need 1,000 mg of calcium and children need 800 to 1,300 mg every day. Broccoli has almost as much calcium as milk. If you add in plain yogurt, you'll double the calcium in this delicious snack.

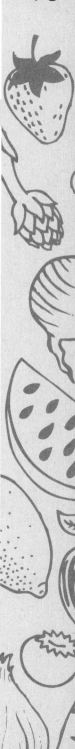

Sweet Potato Smack

Prep time: About 2 min • **Juicing time:** 2 min • **Yield:** 1 serving

Ingredients	Directions
½ lemon	**1** Peel the half lemon, leaving the white pith on.
2 carrots	
1 long, lean sweet potato	**2** Peel the potato. Cut the potato, cabbage, and apple if necessary to fit the juicer feed tube.
¼ green cabbage	
1 apple	**3** Turn on the juicer and place a jug under the spout.
2 teaspoons sesame seeds	**4** Working on a slow speed, process the lemon.
	5 Increase the speed to medium and process the carrots, sweet potato, cabbage, and apple.
	6 Stir the drink, pour into 2 glasses, garnish each with sesame seeds, and enjoy!

Per serving: Calories 162 (From Fat 18); Fat 2g (Saturated 0g); Cholesterol 0mg; Sodium 49mg; Carbohydrate 36g (Dietary Fiber 9g); Protein 4g.

Making Digestive and After-Dinner Juices

When your digestive system is working well, all is well in your body. Digestion starts in your mouth with chewing and breaking down the food. Drinking juice gives you a jump on this first step because the fiber is already separated from the liquid in fruits and vegetables.

You can move your digestion along by drinking vegetables and herbs that assist the liver and gall bladder to provide bile. As anyone with a dysfunctional gall bladder can attest, eating food without enough bile can be painful.

You also can replenish the friendly bacteria that live in your gut by eating one serving (½ cup) of yogurt or kefir three or four times a day for about a week. If you've been taking antibacterial medications, they'll have wiped out the good bacteria along with the bad, and a natural way to get them working for you again is to take acidophilus tablets or natural live yogurt.

Yogurt: The essential stomach food

Probiotics are live microbial organisms that are naturally present in the digestive tract. They help break down your food, but they're also believed to improve immunity, keep the digestive tract intact, and help produce vitamin K. People need these friendly, microscopic critters!

Probiotic yogurt is yogurt that has been made with and still contains a large number of live bacteria. Friendly bacteria such as *Lactobacillus delbrueckii, Lactobacillus acidophilus, Lactobacillus casei, Bifidobacteria,* and *Streptococcus lactis* can help repopulate the friendly microorganisms in your gut, returning it to a healthy condition.

When the friendly bacteria are wiped out by inadequate amount of fiber in the diet, oral antibiotics, infant formula feeding, or toxins in foods such as mercury in fish, less healthy bacteria can move in and thrive. These unhealthy bacteria and yeasts increase the risk of infectious diarrhea and bladder or vaginal yeast infections.

Eating or drinking probiotic yogurt or kefir is one of the best ways to keep your gut and intestines populated with friendly bacteria. But probiotic yogurt will be helpful in supporting your immune system and reducing the risk of other conditions as well, including diarrhea caused by antibiotic use, traveler's diarrhea, side effects of radiation therapy, irritable bowel syndrome, vaginal yeast infections, ulcerative colitis, and Crohn's disease.

By keeping healthy numbers of friendly bacteria in your body, you make it inhospitable and hard for disease-causing bacteria, yeasts, fungi, and parasites to muscle in.

Tummy Tamer

Prep time: About 2 min • **Juicing time:** 2 min • **Yield:** 2 servings

Ingredients	Directions
½ **lemon**	*1* Peel the lemon, leaving the white pith on.
4 **celery stalks**	
3 **carrots**	*2* Cut the pear and the fennel bulb if necessary to fit the juicer feed tube.
1 **pear**	
½ **fennel bulb, stems and leaves intact**	*3* Turn on the juicer and place a jug under the spout.
1 **teaspoon ground fennel seeds**	*4* Working on a slow speed, process the lemon.
	5 Increase the speed to medium and process the celery, carrots, pear, and fennel bulb.
	6 Stir the drink, pour into 2 glasses, garnish each with fennel seeds, and enjoy!

Per serving: Calories 123 (From Fat 8); Fat 1g (Saturated 0g); Cholesterol 0mg; Sodium 157mg; Carbohydrate 30g (Dietary Fiber 3g); Protein 3g.

Amazing Aperitif

Prep time: About 2 min • **Juicing time:** 2 min • **Yield:** 4 servings

Ingredients	Directions
2 medium tomatoes	*1* Peel the lemon, leaving the white pith on.
½ lemon	
2 celery stalks	*2* Cut the zucchini, fennel bulb, and beet if necessary to fit the juicer feed tube.
1 zucchini	
½ English cucumber	*3* Turn on the juicer and place a jug under the spout.
¼ fennel bulb, stems and leaves intact	*4* Working on a slow speed, process the tomatoes and lemon.
1 beet	
1 piece (1-inch) peeled ginger	*5* Increase the speed to medium and process the celery, zucchini, cucumber, and fennel bulb.
½ teaspoon ground fennel seeds	
¼ teaspoon ground licorice root	*6* Increase the speed to high and process the beet and ginger.
¼ teaspoon ground cumin	*7* Stir the fennel seeds, licorice, and cumin into the drink, Pour into 2 glasses, garnish each with fennel seeds, and enjoy!
Whole fennel seeds	

Per serving: *Calories 46 (From Fat 5); Fat 1g (Saturated 0g); Cholesterol 0mg; Sodium 57mg; Carbohydrate 10g (Dietary Fiber 1g); Protein 2g.*

Tip: Look for ground licorice root in health food stores.

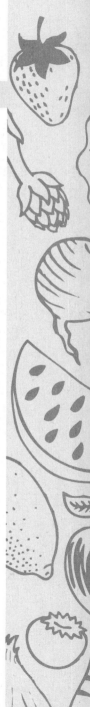

Cabbage Patch

Prep time: About 2 min • **Juicing time:** 2 min • **Yield:** 2 servings

Ingredients	Directions
½ lemon	**1** Peel the lemon, leaving the white pith on.
2 carrots	
½ green cabbage	**2** Cut the cabbage, apple, and fennel bulb if necessary to fit the juicer feed tube.
1 apple	
½ fennel bulb, stems and leaves intact	**3** Turn on the juicer and place a jug under the spout.
1 piece (1-inch) peeled ginger	**4** Working on a slow speed, process the lemon.
¼ cup plain yogurt	**5** Increase the speed to medium and process the carrots, cabbage, apple, fennel bulb, and ginger.
	6 Stir the yogurt into the drink. Pour into 2 glasses, garnish each with fennel seeds, and enjoy!

Per serving: Calories 149 (From Fat 13); Fat 2g (Saturated 0g); Cholesterol 2mg; Sodium 85mg; Carbohydrate 33g (Dietary Fiber 9g); Protein 6g.

Cucumber Chiller

Prep time: About 2 min • **Juicing time:** 2 min • **Yield:** 2 servings

Ingredients	Directions
1 lime	*1* Peel the lime, leaving the white pith on.
3 or 4 sprigs fresh peppermint	
1 English cucumber	*2* Cut the pepper and apples if necessary to fit the juicer feed tube.
½ red pepper	
2 apples	*3* Turn on the juicer and place a jug under the spout.
1 teaspoon ground fennel seeds	*4* Working on a slow speed, process the lime, peppermint, and cucumber, using the cucumber to push the peppermint through the feed tube.
2 sprigs fresh basil	
	5 Increase the speed to medium and process the pepper and apples.
	6 Stir the fennel seeds into the drink. Pour into 2 glasses, garnish each with basil, and enjoy!

Per serving: Calories 129 (From Fat 11); Fat 1g (Saturated 0g); Cholesterol 0mg; Sodium 8mg; Carbohydrate 32g (Dietary Fiber 3g); Protein 2g.

Tip: As a palate cleanser, this juice is the best. Serve it on ice or freeze it slightly and serve with a spoon as a between-course cleanser. Use more or less peppermint as your taste dictates.

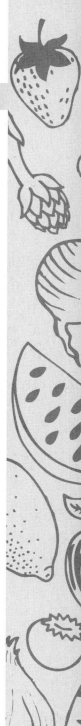

Getting Energized with Exercise Juices

Juice is an excellent pre- or post-exercise drink because, along with the refreshing water, come minerals and vitamins. But you can design these juice drinks so that they're part of your exercise toolkit.

Athletes involved in hard exercise may require higher amounts of potassium-rich foods because potassium works with sodium to maintain the body's water balance. Tomatoes, carrots, celery, spinach, molasses, and unsalted nuts are good sources (300 mg or more) of potassium.

Along with a long list of healing properties, turmeric has one thing to offer people who are exercising: It reduces post-exercise pain by reducing inflammation.

Start soft and finish hard

Prepare for juicing by cleaning, seeding (when necessary), peeling (when necessary), and chopping all your ingredients before you start to juice. Line up the ingredients for juicing in order from soft to hard, because it's easier on you and your juicer if you work in an organized way from easiest (soft) to most difficult (hard).

If you have a multispeed juicer, you can start juicing at the lower speed and gradually increase the speed to match the firmness of the fruit or vegetable. You start on low because the liquid in a soft fruit or vegetable is easier to extract than that of a hard one. The cellulose isn't as strong, so the basket on the juicer isn't required to spin as fast. And if you use a slow speed for soft items, you'll extract more juice from them because, at a high speed, they fly right through the blades and much of the juice remains intact in the pulp. In contrast, for hard vegetables like beets and rutabaga, you need a higher speed to cut through the denser flesh and you need the faster spinning basket to extract the juice from the fiber.

Potassium Power

Prep time: About 3 min • **Juicing time:** 2 min • **Yield:** 2 servings

Ingredients	Directions
3 medium tomatoes	*1* Cut the tomatoes and apple if necessary to fit the juicer feed tube.
½ cup spinach	
2 celery stalks	*2* Turn on the juicer and place a jug under the spout.
2 carrots	
1 apple	*3* Working on a slow speed, process the tomatoes and spinach, alternating them to help push the spinach leaves through.
½ to 1 teaspoon ground turmeric	
2 teaspoons finely chopped walnuts	*4* Increase the speed to medium and process the celery, carrots, and apple.
	5 Stir the turmeric into the drink. Pour into 2 glasses, garnish each with walnuts, and enjoy!

Per serving: Calories 146 (From Fat 27); Fat 3g (Saturated 0g); Cholesterol 0mg; Sodium 104mg; Carbohydrate 31g (Dietary Fiber 3g); Protein 4g.

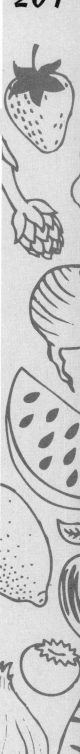

Exercise Elixir

Prep time: About 3 min • **Juicing time:** 2 min • **Yield:** 2 servings

Ingredients	Directions
2 medium tomatoes	*1* Cut the tomatoes and apple if necessary to fit the juicer feed tube.
1 cup packed spinach	
1 handful green beans	*2* Turn on the juicer and place a jug under the spout.
1 small zucchini	
1 apple	*3* Working on a slow speed, process the tomatoes, spinach, and beans.
1 piece (1-inch) peeled ginger	
¼ teaspoon ground turmeric	*4* Increase the speed to medium and process the zucchini, apple, and ginger.
2 teaspoons sesame seeds	
	5 Stir the turmeric into the drink. Pour into 2 glasses, garnish each with sesame seeds, and enjoy!

Per serving: Calories 110 (From Fat 20); Fat 2g (Saturated 0g); Cholesterol 0mg; Sodium 30mg; Carbohydrate 23g (Dietary Fiber 3g); Protein 4g.

Trying Antioxidant Juices

Truth be told, everyone is rusting from the inside out! Oxidation from free radicals is damaging your cells and aging your body. But there is help in slowing down the ravaging oxidants. Antioxidant foods rid the body of these free radicals and keep you safe from their damaging effects.

Top antioxidant vegetables include kale, spinach, Brussels sprouts, alfalfa sprouts, broccoli, beets, red peppers, and eggplant. Toss in antioxidant-rich herbs like thyme and rosemary or sage and oregano, and you have the fixin's for the fountain of youth.

Use fresh herbs

I'm a culinary herbalist, which means that I've studied growing and using herbs, as well as the medicinal benefits of herbs, and I use that knowledge in cooking. This is the way that ancient Greek, Chinese, and Indian healers used herbs — as preventive medicine in foods.

Smoothies are a perfect way to enjoy herbs. Just be sure to use only fresh herbs — dried herbs don't have any of the medicinal values noted here:

✔ **Alfalfa:** High in chlorophyll, nourishes cells

✔ **Basil:** Antidepressant, soothing, relieves indigestion

✔ **Garlic:** Antioxidant, anti-cancer, thins blood, lowers cholesterol

✔ **Lemon balm:** Antioxidant, relaxes, stimulates bile for digestion, antihistamine, antidepressant

✔ **Parsley:** Antioxidant, high in chlorophyll, tonic

✔ **Peppermint:** Soothing, digestive tonic, relieves pain

✔ **Rosemary:** Antioxidant, antiseptic, soothing, anti-inflammatory

✔ **Sage:** Antioxidant, antibiotic, anti-inflammatory

One or two large leaves (for example, of basil or dandelion) or a few smaller leaves (for example, of mint, oregano, or thyme) are blended right in with smoothie recipes.

Ageless Elixir

Prep time: About 3 min • **Juicing time:** 2 min • **Yield:** 2 servings

Ingredients	Directions
2 apples	*1* Cut the apples if necessary to fit the juicer feed tube.
2 broccoli spears	
1 cup coarsely chopped cabbage	*2* Cut the broccoli if necessary to fit the juicer feed tube.
1 cup coarsely chopped kale	*3* Turn on the juicer and place a jug under the spout.
3 to 6 sprigs fresh thyme	*4* Working on a slow speed, process the apples, cabbage, kale, and thyme.
¼ teaspoon minced fresh rosemary, optional	
	5 Increase the speed to medium and process the broccoli.
	6 Stir the rosemary into the drink, pour into 2 glasses, and enjoy.

Per serving: Calories 130 (From Fat 7); Fat 1g (Saturated 0g); Cholesterol 0mg; Sodium 31mg; Carbohydrate 32g (Dietary Fiber 1g); Protein 3g.

Anti-Aging Elixir

Prep time: About 3 min • **Juicing time:** 2 min • **Yield:** 2 servings

Ingredients	Directions
1 orange	*1* Peel the orange and lemon, leaving the white pith on.
½ lemon	
½ red pepper	*2* Cut the broccoli and beet if necessary to fit the juicer feed tube.
2 celery stalks	
1 cup Brussels sprouts	*3* Turn on the juicer and place a jug under the spout.
3 broccoli spears	
1 beet	*4* Working on a slow speed, process the orange and lemon.
¼ teaspoon hot pepper seeds	
	5 Increase the speed to medium and process the red pepper, celery, Brussels sprouts, and broccoli.
	6 Increase the speed to high and process the beet.
	7 Stir the hot pepper seeds into the drink, pour into 2 glasses, and enjoy!

Per serving: Calories 101 (From Fat 6); Fat 1g (Saturated 0g); Cholesterol 0mg; Sodium 109mg; Carbohydrate 23g (Dietary Fiber 3g); Protein 5g.

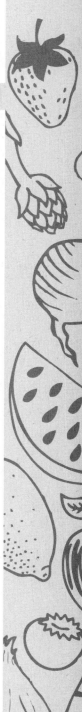

Green Goodness

Prep time: About 3 min • **Juicing time:** 2 min • **Yield:** 2 servings

Ingredients	Directions
1 cup coarsely chopped kale	**1** Peel the half lemon, leaving the white pith on.
3 to 6 sprigs fresh thyme	
½ cup alfalfa sprouts	**2** Cut the broccoli and apple if necessary to fit the juicer feed tube.
½ lemon	
1 zucchini	**3** Turn on the juicer and place a jug under the spout.
2 celery stalks	
2 broccoli spears	**4** Working on a slow speed, process the kale, thyme, alfalfa sprouts, lemon, and zucchini.
1 apple	
¼ teaspoon minced fresh rosemary	**5** Increase the speed to medium and process the celery, broccoli, and apple.
	6 Stir the rosemary into the drink, pour into 2 glasses, and enjoy.

Per serving: Calories 148 (From Fat 14); Fat 1g (Saturated 0g); Cholesterol 0mg; Sodium 123mg; Carbohydrate 32g (Dietary Fiber 4g); Protein 9g.

Tip: Depending on the variety of thyme you use, it may have lots of *thymol,* a healing essential oil that can be pungent but high in antioxidants. Use less thyme if you want.

Keeping Everything Moving with Elimination Juices

Sometimes nature needs a friendly intervention. For those times when nothing is moving, make up a glass of one of these juices and all will soon be well. These recipes can help you in the bathroom department when your body needs a little urging.

One of the best natural laxatives is the prune. Eat it stewed, drink the juice, or eat the dried form for relief from constipation. Prunes are rich in antioxidants, vitamin A, potassium, iron, and dietary fiber — that's why I use them whole in these drinks. Prunes also feed the friendly bacteria in the digestive tract for extra moving power.

Spice it up!

Most spices have medicinal value and, for that reason, they're welcome in smoothies. But unless you add spices in medicinal doses (usually 1 to 3 teaspoons), don't expect that they'll do all they can for your body. Still, they're a healthy way to bring out the flavors of smoothies. Here are some of the most popular spices that jazz up smoothies and their medicinal values:

✔ **Cayenne:** Tonic, antiseptic, aids blood circulation and elimination

✔ **Cinnamon:** Aids digestion, nausea, vomiting, diarrhea; calms stomach pain

✔ **Clove:** Antioxidant, anesthetic, fights fungal infection

✔ **Echinacea:** Stimulates immune system, anti-inflammatory, antiseptic, lymph tonic

✔ **Fennel:** Soothing digestive, anti-inflammatory

✔ **Ginger:** Anti-nausea, relieves headache and arthritis

✔ **Licorice:** Tonic, anti-inflammatory, antibacterial

✔ **Turmeric:** Antioxidant, antiviral, anti-inflammatory

In my recipes, I recommend adding between ⅛ and ¼ teaspoon of ground spices for every one or two servings. If you're using a tincture, follow directions for the number of drops; ½ to 1 garlic clove is pretty strong; a ½-inch piece of candied ginger in smoothies is warming. A good rule to follow is to start with a small amount, taste, and add more if you want.

Prune Power

Prep time: About 2 min • **Juicing time:** 2 min • **Yield:** 1 serving

Ingredients	Directions
1 black plum	**1** Cut the plum in half and remove the stones.
1 carrot	
1 celery stalk	**2** Cut the beet if necessary to fit the juicer feed tube.
1 beet	**3** Turn on the juicer and place a jug under the spout.
¼ cup chopped prunes	
1 teaspoon apple cider vinegar	**4** Working on a slow speed, process the plum.
¼ teaspoon ground licorice	**5** Increase the speed to medium and process the carrot and celery.
	6 Increase the speed to high and process the beet.
	7 Combine the vegetable juice, the prunes, cider vinegar, and licorice in a blender jug and process on high for 30 seconds or until smooth. Pour into a glass and stay close to home!

Per serving: Calories 212 (From Fat 9); Fat 1g (Saturated 0g); Cholesterol 0mg; Sodium 143mg; Carbohydrate 52g (Dietary Fiber 4g); Protein 4g.

Tip: Take this slow and easy. A small glass to start may be enough. If not, drink another small glass and wait a couple hours. This is powerful stuff!

Dynamite Dandelion

Prep time: About 2 min • **Juicing time:** 2 min • **Yield:** 1 serving

Ingredients	Directions
1 cup fresh dandelion leaves or spinach	**1** Cut the apple and beet if necessary to fit the juicer feed tube.
1 celery stalk	
1 apple	**2** Turn on the juicer and place a jug under the spout.
1 beet	
1 teaspoon ground dandelion root	**3** Working on a slow speed, process the dandelion leaves and celery, pushing through the leaves with the celery.
¼ teaspoon ground licorice	
	4 Increase the speed to medium and process the apple.
	5 Increase the speed to high and process the beet.
	6 Stir the dandelion root powder and ground licorice into the drink. Pour into 2 glasses and stay close to home!

Per serving: Calories 152 (From Fat 10); Fat 1g (Saturated 0g); Cholesterol 0mg; Sodium 161mg; Carbohydrate 36g (Dietary Fiber 3g); Protein 4g.

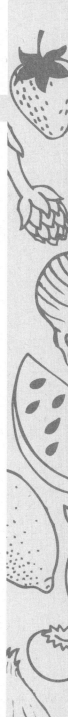

Rocking the Party: Vegetable Mocktails and Cocktail Mixers

Vegetable juice makes a great drink anytime, anywhere, but when you have to drive or you just don't want the alcohol, they're a satisfying alternative.

When you *are* drinking alcohol, sometimes only savory will do. When sweet drinks just aren't satisfying enough, vegetable juices can step up and form the basis for really creative cocktails. (As always, the alcohol is optional.) These recipes are great, no matter the occasion.

Noting some great vegetable mixers

Vegetables are a natural mixer for drinks. Here are some excellent choices:

✔ **Carrot:** Because of their natural sweetness, carrots make a great mixer for most of the following vegetables. Use them with vodka, rye, or rum.

✔ **Celery:** Celery juice can be strong, so always mix it with other vegetables such as cucumbers, tomatoes, and fennel. Mix with vodka, Scotch, or rum.

✔ **Cucumbers:** Use chilled cucumber juice to mix with vodka and tonic or soda for a refreshing and light summer cooler.

✔ **Fennel:** With its light anise flavor, the juice from fennel bulb mixes well with other vegetable juice and ground cumin or coriander for a mix for vodka or gin.

✔ **Peppers:** Red or green bell peppers are best if mixed with other vegetables such as tomatoes and cucumber or fennel, and they're robust enough to use with Scotch or rum.

✔ **Tomatoes:** They're juicy and mild in flavor, so mix with cucumber or even onion for a more robust mixer to use with vodka or rye.

✔ **Zucchini:** The flavor is very mild and it mixes well with most vegetable juice such as carrot or beet. If combined in a vegetable mix, you can use it with vodka or rye.

Vegetable Mocktail

Prep time: 4 minutes • **Juicing time:** 2 min • **Yield:** 4 servings

Ingredients	Directions
4 medium tomatoes	**1** Cut the tomatoes, pepper, fennel, and apple if necessary to fit the juicer feed tube.
3 sprigs parsley	
½ red bell pepper	**2** Turn on the juicer and place a jug under the spout.
2 carrots	
2 celery stalks	**3** Working on a slow speed, process the tomatoes and parsley.
¼ fennel bulb, stem and leaves intact	
1 apple	**4** Increase the speed to medium and process the pepper, celery, fennel, and apple.
¼ teaspoon ground cumin	
¼ teaspoon hot pepper flakes	**5** Stir the cumin, pepper flakes, Worcestershire sauce, and salt into the drink. Pour into 2 glasses, garnish with basil, and enjoy!
Dash Worcestershire sauce	
Pinch coarse sea salt	
2 sprigs basil	

Per serving: *Calories 78 (From Fat 8); Fat 1g (Saturated 0g); Cholesterol 0mg; Sodium 87mg; Carbohydrate 18g (Dietary Fiber 1g); Protein 2g.*

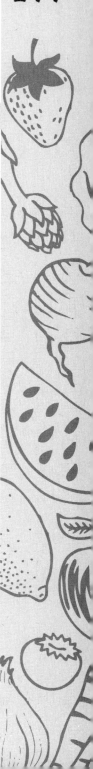

Italian Vegetable Mocktail

Prep time: About 3 min • **Juicing time:** 2 min • **Yield:** 2 servings

Ingredients	Directions
2 medium tomatoes	*1* Cut the tomatoes, eggplant, zucchini, and apple if necessary to fit the juicer feed tube.
1 clove garlic, optional	
3 sprigs fresh oregano	*2* Turn on the juicer and place a jug under the spout.
1 baby eggplant	
2 small zucchini	*3* Working on a slow speed, process the tomatoes, garlic, oregano, and eggplant, pushing the oregano through the feed tube with the eggplant.
2 celery stalks	
1 apple	
¼ teaspoon chopped fresh thyme or a pinch chopped fresh rosemary	*4* Increase the speed to medium and process the zucchini, celery, apple, and ginger.
¼ teaspoon coarse sea salt	*5* Stir the thyme, rosemary, and salt into the drink. Pour into 2 glasses, garnish with basil, and enjoy!
2 sprigs fresh basil	

Per serving: Calories 99 (From Fat 13); Fat 1g (Saturated 0g); Cholesterol 0mg; Sodium 276mg; Carbohydrate 21g (Dietary Fiber 6g); Protein 5g.

Fiery Red Mixer

Prep time: About 3 min • **Juicing time:** 2 min • **Yield:** 2 servings

Ingredients	Directions
2 oranges	**1** Peel the oranges and lime, leaving the white pith on.
1 lime	
½ red bell pepper	**2** Cut the pepper and beets if necessary to fit the feed tube of the juicer.
1 celery stalk	
2 carrots	**3** Turn on the juicer and place a jug under the spout.
2 beets	
1 piece (1-inch) peeled fresh ginger	**4** Working on a slow speed, process the oranges and lime.
Dash hot sauce	**5** Increase the speed to medium and process the pepper, celery, and carrots.
Pinch coarse sea salt	
2 ounces vodka, rum, or gin	**6** Increase the speed to high and process the beets and ginger.
2 green onions	
	7 Stir the cumin, hot sauce, salt, and alcohol into the juice. Pour into 2 glasses, garnish each with green onion, and enjoy!

Per serving: Calories 207 (From Fat 5); Fat 1g (Saturated 0g); Cholesterol 0mg; Sodium 161mg; Carbohydrate 34g (Dietary Fiber 4g); Protein 4g.

Tip: Serve this drink neat or over ice.

Tip: Try rimming the glass with herbed salt. In a saucer, combine ¼ cup coarse sea salt, 1 teaspoon fresh or dried thyme, and ½ teaspoon fresh or dried rosemary. Run a wedge of lime around the edges of the glasses to wet the rims and tip the rims into the salt mixture. Twist the glasses to coat the rims evenly with the herbed salt mixture.

Vary It: For the very daring, spice up this red-hot mixer by adding a whole hot chile pepper.

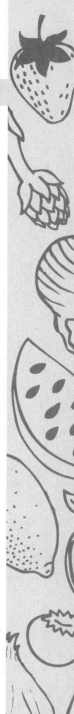

Gingered Citrus Mixer

Prep time: About 6 min • **Juicing time:** 2 min • **Yield:** 2 servings

Ingredients	Directions
1 honeydew melon	**1** Cut the melon in half. Scoop out the seeds and trim away the rind from each half. Discard the seeds and rind. Cut the flesh into wedges to fit the juicer feed tube.
2 oranges	
3 sprigs fresh basil	
1 lime	**2** Peel the oranges and lime, leaving the white pith on.
2 celery stalks	
2 carrots	**3** Turn on the juicer and place a jug under the spout.
1 piece (2-inches) peeled fresh ginger	**4** Working on a slow speed, process the melon, oranges, basil, and lime.
2 ounces vodka, rum, gin per serving	**5** Increase the speed to medium and process the celery, carrots, and ginger.
	6 Stir the alcohol into the juice, pour into 2 glasses, and enjoy!

Per serving Calories 429 (From Fat 2); Fat 0g (Saturated 0g); Cholesterol 0mg; Sodium 266mg; Carbohydrate 93g (Dietary Fiber 2g); Protein 8g.

Chapter 14

Recycling Your Juicing Leftovers

In This Chapter

▶ Thinking ahead

▶ Using pulp for masks and scrubs

▶ Trying some recipes using the pulp

Recipes in This Chapter

⟳ Apple Carrot Muffins

▶ Ginger Beet Soup

▶ Quinoa Salad

⟳ Mediterranean Tomato Sauce

▶ Red Pepper Curry Sauce

⟳ Fruit Syrup

⟳ Fruit Cobbler

🍸 🍲 ⟳ 🍴 🥄 🌿

The amount of pulp you produce will astound you the first time you fire up the juicer and make yourself a fresh juice. For every serving of juice, you accumulate 3 to 4 cups of pulp. Of course, you can dump the mountain of pulp and go on your way. But think of the investment you've made in fruits and vegetables for juicing. You don't want to let part of that precious food — and all those vitamins, minerals, phytonutrients, and fiber — go to waste.

If you want to get the full benefit from the nutrients in whole fruits or vegetables, you have to find a way to eat the pulp as well as drink the juice.

Why not think of the by-product of juicing as an opportunity to add nutrients and valuable fiber to your favorite recipes? With a little forethought, you can separate the pulp by fruit and vegetable and freeze it for use in all kinds of recipes — from soups to sauces to dips and spreads and baked goods. You can even make masks, scrubs, and other spa-type beauty products with it. In this chapter, I show you how to make quick work of dealing with the pulp from the fruits and vegetables you juice.

Planning Ahead

You need to think about how you'll use the pulp before you start to juice. Let's say you want to make your favorite bran muffin recipe and you plan to add pulp to the recipe for the benefit of nutrients and flavor. Sounds good. But what if you don't feel like a fruit juice? Many vegetables can be added to sweet baked goods, but other vegetables don't work as well.

Mostly this is a matter of common sense and experimentation: Mild-tasting vegetables — like beets, carrots, and zucchini — can be added to the batter of cookies, breads, muffins, and other sweet baked goods without adversely affecting the flavor. On the other hand, strong-tasting vegetables — like onions, cabbage, and garlic — aren't appropriate for baked goods. You can use those stronger-tasting vegetables in soups, sauces, dips, and other savory dishes.

Save the plastic bags that you get in the produce section of your supermarket, and use them to line the pulp container of your juicer before you start juicing. Because produce bags are thin, they won't interfere with the fit of the pulp container into the juicer. The added bonus is that you don't have to wash the pulp container — just lift out the bag!

Juice the vegetables you want to add to a recipe first. Stop the juicer, remove the bag with the pulp, label it, and either refrigerate or freeze it. Reline the pulp container with a new produce bag and continue to juice the remaining ingredients.

If you'll be saving pulp for another recipe, be sure to remove the core, seeds, or pith before juicing.

Pulp is liquid-free fresh fruits or vegetables. Because it's fresh, it spoils quickly, so it must be used immediately or frozen for later use. If you're planning to make a recipe using the pulp right away, you can seal the bag of pulp and keep it in the refrigerator for up to three days. If you know you won't be using the pulp right away, transfer the pulp to a zip-top freezer bag, label and force the air out of the freezer bag, seal the top, and freeze for up to three months.

Measure 1 cup, 2 cups, or 4 cups of pulp into a freezer bag before labeling and freezing it. This will give you pre-measured amounts for your recipes.

Recycling Pulp

If you think about how you'll use the pulp and plan ahead, there is no reason why you can't use it all in everyday recipes. I've added onion and apple pulp to my Thanksgiving turkey dressing, and I've beefed up homemade or store-bought tzatziki dip with cucumber or zucchini pulp. Sometimes carrots and celery end up in the dip, but that only adds color along with the nutrients I don't want to waste. You can even pop frozen pulp right into a cooking soup or stew. The only limit is your imagination! In this section, I give you some recipes to get you started.

Apple Carrot Muffins

Prep time: About 15 min • **Cooking time:** 25 min • **Yield:** 12 muffins

Ingredients	Directions
⅔ **cup buttermilk**	*1* Line a 12-cup muffin pan with paper or silicone liners and preheat the oven to 400°F.
¼ **cup canola oil**	
1 large egg	*2* In a bowl, whisk together the buttermilk, oil, and egg. Stir in the apple and carrot pulp. Set aside.
¾ **cup apple pulp (about 5 apples juiced)**	
¾ **cup carrot pulp (about 4 large carrots juiced)**	*3* In a large bowl, combine the bran cereal, flour, sugar, baking soda, cinnamon, salt, and almonds. Stir well with a fork to mix.
1¾ **cups bran cereal**	
1¼ **cups all-purpose flour**	*4* Stir the buttermilk mixture into the flour mixture until moistened. Spoon into the lined muffin tin cups until about three-quarters full.
⅔ **cup lightly packed brown sugar**	
1¼ **teaspoons baking soda**	*5* Bake for 20 to 25 minutes or until a toothpick comes out clean when inserted into the center of a muffin. Cool the muffins in the pan and remove to a cooling rack to cool completely.
¾ **teaspoon ground cinnamon**	
¼ **teaspoon salt**	
¼ **cup chopped almonds**	

Per serving: *Calories 181 (From Fat 59); Fat 7g (Saturated 227g); Cholesterol 18mg; Sodium 227mg; Carbohydrate 30g (Dietary Fiber 4g); Protein 4g.*

Vary It: You can use the pulp from parsnips, rutabaga, turnip, carrots, celery, and almost any fruit, or a combination of any of these. Try pineapple in place of the apple.

Tip: If you don't have pulp, you can still make this recipe by using ¾ cup shredded apple and ¾ cup shredded carrot.

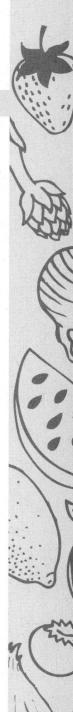

Ginger Beet Soup

Prep time: About 10 min • **Cooking time:** 25 min • **Yield:** 4 servings

Ingredients	Directions
2 tablespoons olive oil 1 onion, chopped	*1* In a saucepan over medium-high heat, heat the oil. Sauté the onion for 5 minutes.
1 leek, white part only, sliced 1 clove garlic, minced	*2* Add the leek and garlic and cook, stirring frequently for 3 to 4 minutes or until soft.
3 cups chicken or beef broth 2 cups chopped beets 2 cups beet or beet-vegetable pulp (6 to 8 beets juiced)	*3* Add the broth, increase the heat to high, and bring to a boil. Add the beets, cover, reduce the heat, and simmer for 20 minutes.
1 tablespoon soy sauce 1 piece (1-inch) fresh ginger, minced	*4* Stir in the pulp, soy sauce, and ginger. Reduce the heat to medium-low and simmer for 15 minutes or until the beets and beet pulp are soft.
2 green onions, sliced in half lengthwise	*5* Ladle into bowls and garnish each with a green onion half.

Per serving: Calories 163 (From Fat 91); Fat 10g (Saturated 2g); Cholesterol 4mg; Sodium 1,052mg; Carbohydrate 16g (Dietary Fiber 4g); Protein 4g.

Tip: If the vegetable pulp you're using has some ginger in it, don't add the fresh ginger as directed in the recipe.

Tip: The soy sauce adds salt naturally, but you can taste the soup and add salt to your preference.

Vary It: If you have beet pulp mixed with other vegetables and even some fruit, use it in this soup. Orange and apple give a pleasingly sweet note to the recipe.

Quinoa Salad

Prep time: About 15 min • **Cooking time:** 15 min • **Yield:** 6 servings

Ingredients	Directions
2 cups vegetable or chicken broth 1 cup quinoa, rinsed and drained ¼ cup extra-virgin olive oil	**1** In a saucepan, bring broth to a boil over high heat. Add the quinoa, stir, and bring to a light boil. Reduce heat to medium-low and simmer for 15 minutes or until the liquid is absorbed. Remove from the burner and set aside to cool.
3 tablespoons freshly squeezed lemon juice 2 tablespoons chopped fresh basil	**2** Meanwhile, in a glass jar with a tight-fitting lid, combine the oil, lemon juice, and basil. Shake well and set aside to use as the dressing.
2 cups vegetable pulp ½ red onion, chopped Sea salt and pepper to taste ½ cup chopped almonds	**3** In a bowl, toss the quinoa with the vegetable pulp and red onion. Drizzle the dressing over and toss well to coat the ingredients. Grind the sea salt over the salad, taste, and add more if necessary. Garnish with almonds.

Per serving: Calories 274 (From Fat 142); Fat 16g (Saturated 2g); Cholesterol 0mg; Sodium 419mg; Carbohydrate 27g (Dietary Fiber 12g); Protein 7g.

Vary It: You can use the pulp from any of the following vegetable juice recipes (all in Chapter 13): Beet in Motion, Brassy Brassica, Waldorf Salad, Winter Roots, Smokin' Peppers, Healthy Giant, Seed Power, and any others with vegetables that you would like to try in the salad.

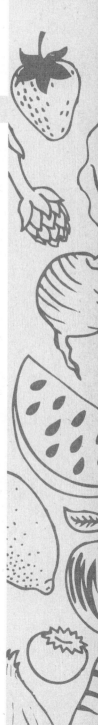

Mediterranean Tomato Sauce

Prep time: About 10 min • **Cooking time:** 25 min • **Yield:** 6 servings

Ingredients	Directions
2 tablespoons olive oil	*1* In a saucepan over medium-high heat, heat the oil. Sauté the onion for 5 minutes.
1 onion, chopped	
2 cloves garlic, minced	*2* Add the garlic and cook, stirring frequently, for 2 minutes or until soft.
2 cups tomato-vegetable pulp (see Vary It!)	
One 28-ounce can whole tomatoes with juice	*3* Add the pulp and tomatoes and their juice. Increase heat to high and bring to a boil.
2 tablespoons red wine vinegar	*4* Stir in the vinegar, basil, and oregano. Press tomatoes with the back of a wooden spoon to break them up. Reduce the heat to medium-low and simmer for 15 minutes or until the sauce reaches the desired thickness.
2 tablespoons chopped fresh basil	
1 tablespoon chopped fresh oregano	

Per serving: Calories 78 (From Fat 43); Fat 5g (Saturated 1g); Cholesterol 0mg; Sodium 197mg; Carbohydrate 9g (Dietary Fiber 3g); Protein 2g.

Tip: To make chicken Parmesan, in a casserole dish, spoon 2 cups Mediterranean Tomato Sauce over four boneless, skinless chicken breasts. Grate Parmesan cheese over the top, cover with a lid or foil, and bake at 350°F for 35 to 40 minutes or until the juices in the chicken run clear when slit with a knife.

Vary It: You can use the pulp from any of the following vegetable juice recipes (all in Chapter 13): Smokin' Peppers, Healthy Giant, Amazing Aperitif, Potassium Power, Exercise Elixir, Spicy Tomato Mocktail or Italian Vegetable Mocktail.

Red Pepper Curry Sauce

Prep time: About 8 min • **Cooking time:** 25 min • **Yield:** 8 servings

Ingredients	Directions
2 tablespoons olive oil 1 onion, chopped	*1* In a saucepan over medium-high heat, heat the oil. Sauté the onion for 5 minutes.
1 red pepper, chopped 2 cloves garlic, minced 2 teaspoons curry powder	*2* Add the pepper, garlic and curry powder. Cook, stirring frequently for 2 minutes or until vegetables are soft.
½ cup pepper-vegetable pulp (see Vary It!) 1 cup chicken broth	*3* Add the pulp, broth, and vinegar. Increase the heat to high and bring to a boil.
1 tablespoon rice vinegar 1 tablespoon chopped fresh cilantro	*4* Reduce the heat to medium-low and simmer for 15 minutes or until sauce reaches the desired thickness. Remove from the heat and stir in the cilantro.

Per serving: Calories 49 (From Fat 36); Fat 4g (Saturated 1g); Cholesterol 1mg; Sodium 126mg; Carbohydrate 3g (Dietary Fiber 3g); Protein 1g.

Vary It: You can use the pulp from any of the following vegetable juice recipes (all in Chapter 13) to make this zippy sauce: Sunriser, Smokin' Peppers, Anti-Aging Elixir, or Fiery Red Mixer. Use it as a dip for raw or roasted vegetables or drizzle over cooked fish or chicken.

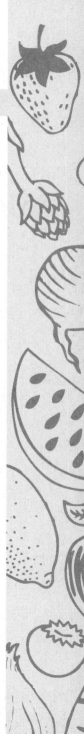

Fruit Syrup

Prep time: About 1 min • **Cooking time:** 15 min • **Yield:** 8 servings

Ingredients	Directions
2 cups water	**1** In a saucepan over medium-high heat, bring the water to a boil.
1 cup granulated sugar	
1 cup fruit pulp	**2** Stir in the sugar. Reduce the heat and simmer, stirring frequently for 12 to 15 minutes or until syrup thickens.
	3 Add the fruit pulp and bring the syrup to a boil.

Per serving: Calories 97 (From Fat 0); Fat 0g (Saturated 0g); Cholesterol 0mg; Sodium 0mg; Carbohydrate 25g (Dietary Fiber 1g); Protein 0g.

Vary It: Use any fruit pulp from the fruit juices in Chapter 12. Try citrus fruit pulp from Sunny Side Up or any of the berry or tropical fruit pulp combinations.

Fruit Cobbler

Prep time: About 8 min • **Cooking time:** 30 min • **Yield:** 6 servings

Ingredients	Directions
4 apples, peeled and sliced 2 cups fruit pulp	*1* Grease a 1½-quart baking dish and preheat the oven to 375°F.
⅓ cup butter 1¼ cups lightly packed brown sugar	*2* Spread the apple slices and pulp evenly over the bottom of the prepared casserole.
⅔ cup old-fashioned rolled oats ⅓ cup all-purpose flour	*3* In a bowl, cream together the butter and the sugar. Add the oats, flour, cinnamon, and salt. Stir until the mixture is crumbly and well mixed.
¼ teaspoon cinnamon ¼ teaspoon salt	*4* Spread the oat mixture evenly over the fruit in the casserole. Bake for 35 minutes or until the apples are tender and the topping is golden brown.

Per serving: Calories 369 (From Fat 98); Fat 11g (Saturated 6g); Cholesterol 27mg; Sodium 117mg; Carbohydrate 69g (Dietary Fiber 4g); Protein 2g.

Vary It: Tree fruits — apples, pears, plums, apricots, peaches, and nectarines — work well in this cobbler. I like to use some fresh apples along with the pulp, especially if there is no apple in the pulp.

Tip: If the fruit pulp is wet, drain it before using it in this recipe.

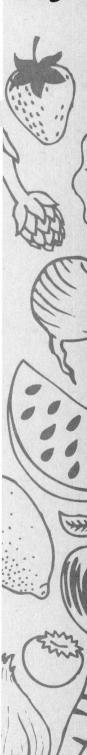

Creating Your Very Own Kitchen Spa with Pulp

Yes, you can use fruit or vegetable pulp for beauty products! Not only does this put to use all those fruits and vegetables, but it also saves you the time and money of going to a spa. And your skin will thank you for it!

Skin-refining face mask

The alpha-hydroxy acids (AHAs) that expensive "natural" skin creams take advantage of are actually found in some of the fruits you use in juicing. The same proteolytic enzymes that play a role in digestion also can be used to soften and "digest" dead skin, leaving your skin feeling smooth and refined.

To make this skin-refining face mask, you need the following:

- ½ cup pineapple, kiwifruit, papaya, and/or mango pulp (You can use just one type of pulp, or a combination, as long as you use ½ cup total.)
- ½ cup plain yogurt, drained

Follow these steps:

1. **In a bowl, combine the ingredients.**
2. **Cover a pillow with a towel, and relax by reclining on a sofa or bed.**
3. **Pat the mixture on your face and neck or, even better, have someone else apply the mixture while you relax.**

   Keep the mixture on your face for ten minutes.
4. **Rinse off using warm water.**

Cooling cucumber eye pack

If you work at a computer all day, you're no stranger to eyestrain. This eye pack is a simple way to cool the stinging and help reduce the swelling and redness that come with overworked eyes.

To make this eye pack, you need the following:

- 2 strips (2 by 6 inches) cotton or cheesecloth
- ¼ cup cucumber pulp
- 2 small zip-top bags

Follow these steps:

1. **Fold each cotton strip in half.**
2. **Divide the cucumber pulp in half and put an equal amount on the center of one side of each cotton strip.**
3. **Pat each pulp mound into an oval shape that is roughly 1½ inches long by 1 inch wide, and fold the strip over so that the mound is covered on both sides by the cotton.**
4. **Place each strip into a bag and freeze the pulp for at least 20 minutes.**
5. **Cover a pillow with a towel, and relax by reclining on a sofa or bed.**
6. **Remove the frozen strips from the bags.**
7. **Close your eyes and place a strip with the frozen cucumber over each eye.**

   Keep the eye packs on for 20 minutes or longer.

You can refreeze the cucumber strips once and reuse them.

Salt scrub

Salt has a skin-softening and rejuvenating effect. You can use this scrub on your hands, feet, body, or face.

To make this scrub, you need the following:

- 1 cup apple, pear, mango, papaya, pineapple, carrot, or cucumber pulp (You can use just one type of pulp, or a combination, as long as you use 1 cup total.)
- 1 cup salt
- 3 tablespoons vegetable oil or almond oil
- 20 to 40 drops essential oil (such as lavender, mint, patchouli, or rose), optional

Follow these steps:

1. **In a bowl, combine the ingredients.**
2. **Transfer the mixture to a clean jar with a lid.**
3. **Use immediately or keep in the refrigerator for up to two weeks.**

Part IV
Blending Fresh Smoothies

Accessing the fiber in smoothies

- ✏ Fruit and vegetable fiber helps you stay healthy because it helps cleanse your bowels and colon.
- ✏ Fiber stays with you longer, giving you a feeling of being full longer.
- ✏ Fiber helps to lower your blood sugar levels.
- ✏ Fiber helps your heart by lowering cholesterol levels.

For some additional dessert smoothie recipes, go to www.dummies.com/extras/juicingsmoothies.

In this part . . .

- ✔ Get the most out of your smoothies by adding super nutritious ingredients and start living healthier.

- ✔ Become blender-savvy and discover the correct order of adding ingredients to the blender so that your smoothies are indeed smooth.

- ✔ Find out how to increase your nutrient intake by widening your list of fruit and vegetable smoothies.

- ✔ Know all about dairy ingredients, including the types of milk and cheeses, to use in smoothies.

- ✔ Make professional iced drinks and frozen treats for everyday drinking or special events where you can impress your friends and stay cool.

Chapter 15

Eyeing Smoothie Ingredients and Techniques

M aking smoothies requires no special equipment that most house-holds don't already have — all you need is a blender. And the wide variety of ingredients that can go into fresh smoothies make them not only healthy but delicious and exciting drinks! In this chapter, I fill you in on the many ingredients that can go into smoothies. Then I explain how to make smoothies — it's as easy as can be.

Identifying Smoothie Ingredients

Building the perfect smoothie isn't hard, especially if you have a wide variety of fruits, vegetables, and other healthy ingredients on hand. Liquids are always included in smoothies and they always go first into the blender. After that, the only thing you need is an imagination and the willingness to try new combinations of ingredients!

Liquids

If you've never made a smoothie before, it may surprise you that juices or other liquids are important components of smoothies. Because smoothies are so thick, you may have thought that they were made only with fruits, vegetables, and some other healthy ingredients.

In fact, the liquid you choose for your smoothie is critical to the actual blending of the drink. It eases the spinning of the blades, enabling the other ingredients to be emulsified. If you like to play with your food, try toying with the amount of liquid you add to see how it changes the consistency of the drink — the more liquid in the smoothie, the thinner it will be.

Of course, liquids add taste and nutrients too, but some add extra calories to the drink, so choosing which liquids to use is as important as choosing which fruits, vegetables, and other ingredients will go into your smoothie.

Here are some liquids you can use in smoothies:

- **Fresh fruit juices:** Freshly squeezed or juiced fruits are better than bottled juices, but both add nutrients and virtually no fat. Fruit juices increase the natural sugars in a smoothie, though. If you have to go with store-bought juices, remember to check the label and avoid those with added sugar, corn syrup, and oil.

- **Coconut water:** High in potassium and electrolytes, it's a great low-calorie, fat-free liquid for smoothies. It's becoming widely available in convenience stores and supermarkets, but some stores still stock it in the international foods aisle or you may find it in Asian markets.

- **Fresh vegetable juices:** Freshly juiced vegetables add nutrients without the fat and excessive sugars. Bottled vegetable juices are convenient but not as nutritious as juicing your own vegetables. If you have to go with store-bought vegetable juice, read the label and avoid those with sugar, preservatives, or high amounts of sodium.

- **Vegetable or chicken broth:** Save vegetable cooking water or chicken broth for vegetable smoothies because this broth contains water-soluble nutrients.

- **Milk:** Lowfat or skim milk adds calcium and protein along with other nutrients to the drink. Use whole milk if you need the extra fat.

- **Milk substitutes:** Coconut, rice, soy, or any of the nut milks make a delicious, nondairy or vegan addition to either fruit or vegetable smoothies.

- **Herb juices:** Green herbs are loaded with antioxidants, vitamins, minerals, chlorophyll, and other phytonutrients, so juice them with fruits or vegetables for use in smoothies.

- **Miscellaneous liquids:** You can add these to any of the liquids listed earlier: freshly brewed, chilled green tea; kombucha (or other seaweed water); noni or acai berry juice; herb juices, tinctures, or *decoctions* (liquids made from pouring boiling water over roots, seeds, and bark); coconut oil, flaxseed oil; or cod liver oil.

Use about ½ cup of liquid per serving for smoothies and always put liquid into the blender first.

Fruits

Not surprisingly, the most common ingredient in smoothies is fruit. The following fruits are great for smoothies:

- Acai berries
- Apples
- Apricots
- Bananas
- Blackberries
- Blueberries
- Cherries
- Grapefruit
- Guava
- Kiwifruit
- Lemons
- Limes
- Mangoes
- Oranges
- Papaya
- Peaches
- Pears
- Pineapple
- Plums
- Pomegranates
- Raspberries

Vegetables

Vegetables are full of fiber and incredible phytonutrients, and the added benefit is that most are lower in sugar than fruits. Many people don't think of vegetables when they think of smoothies, but why not use these nutrient-rich and often neglected foods? Here are some vegetables that work well in smoothies:

- Beans
- Beets
- Broccoli
- Brussels sprouts
- Cabbage
- Carrots
- Cauliflower
- Corn
- Kale, spinach, Swiss chard
- Parsnips
- Peas
- Peppers
- Rutabaga
- Squash
- Turnips

 If you find that the taste of vegetables is just not sweet enough, add an apple to sweeten the drink. If that isn't enough, try dates or figs and, as a last resort, add some sweeteners — but keep reducing the amount of fruit or sweetener in subsequent smoothies until you're totally accustomed to the taste of the drink without it.

 Start with vegetables you like. Carrots, peas, and corn are favorite vegetables with children (and many adults) because they're higher in natural sugars. When converting to vegetable smoothies, use them in combination with vegetables that are low in sugar.

Green grasses and sprouts

Ever wonder what animals get from grass? Grass is a rich source of nutrients. As Eastern medicine teaches, humans are wise to imitate their pets and eat or *drink* cereal grasses and algae (also known as green foods) because they're high in chlorophyll.

A natural blood purifier, chlorophyll is important to overall healing. Here's how it works: The blood carries nutrients, phytonutrients, and enzymes, but it also transports anaerobic bacteria, yeast, and fungus. As the immune system attacks these unwanted substances, debris is left in the blood. Chlorophyll cleans out the blood crud that causes cell damage. Chlorophyll not only manages bacterial growth, but is also anti-inflammatory.

Perhaps the least known benefit of green foods is their ability to keep your body's pH balanced. Why is this important? A balanced pH level (slightly alkaline) increases your resistance to disease. All sorts of things like stress, sugar, caffeine, high-protein intake, even rock music can increase your body's pH level, so add the following green grasses and sprouts to smoothies:

- **Cereal grasses:** Barley and wheat grass are high in chlorophyll and contain important enzymes. You can grow and use fresh, young green grasses or purchase them dried and add by the spoonful to smoothies.

- **Microalgae:** Spirulina is rich in chlorophyll, beta-carotene, and the beneficial fatty acid gamma-linolenic acid (GLA). It also has antioxidant and anti-inflammatory properties. Similar to spirulina (except that it contains more chlorophyll and less protein and beta-carotene), chlorella's tough cell wall binds with heavy metals, pesticides, and other carcinogens, helping to rid the body of them.

- **Sprouts:** Bean, broccoli, sunflower, no matter what sprout you opt for, when you eat it, you're consuming the tiny, whole plant including the root, the stem, and the head. All the micronutrients found in the whole plant are available to you, and it's likely that you'll consume a hundred or more mini plants in one smoothie. Adding broccoli sprouts to your smoothies is an easy way to consume significant amounts of cancer-fighting indoles and sulforaphanes.

Seaweed

Each type of seaweed (or sea vegetable) has its own nutrient profile, but as a group they have several things in common:

- They're rich in vitamins, minerals, trace elements, and amino acids (the building blocks of proteins).

- They're particularly good sources of iodine, calcium, and iron.

- They can rid the body of heavy metals and protect against radiation.

- The iodine in seaweed protects against thyroid disease and cancer from atmospheric nuclear dust.

All in all, this is a pretty impressive group of plants that is so easily incorporated into smoothies. Here are some sea vegetables to add to your next drink:

- ✔ **Arame:** Dried and cut into strands, this black, mild seaweed can be softened easily by immersing it in cool water for about 15 minutes before blending in drinks. It's extremely high in iodine (100 to 500 times more than in shellfish), as well as high in iron, vitamin A, and calcium (more than ten times the calcium found in milk).

- ✔ **Kombu:** Sometimes called kelp, this seaweed is often available in flakes, which are easy to add to smoothies before blending. With its potassium, calcium, vitamins A and C, and high iodine, kombu is a great addition to smoothies.

- ✔ **Wakame:** When it grows, this sea vegetable is leathery and deep green in color. It resembles spinach in taste. Soak it in cool water for about ten minutes and chop it before blending into smoothies. Wakame is a good source of protein, iron, calcium, sodium, and vitamins A, C, E, and K.

Both the Canadian Food Inspection Agency (CFIA) and the Food Standards Agency (FSA) in the United Kingdom have issued warnings that hijiki, a brown sea vegetable high in nutrients and widely consumed in Japan, contains inorganic arsenic that can exceed tolerable daily intake levels. This warning sparked debate and controversy. The Japanese Ministry of Health and Welfare stated, "There are no records of cases of arsenic poisoning as a result of the arsenic content of sea vegetables." No definitive answer has been given on this issue, but it's important to choose sea vegetables from distributors you trust that hand-harvest it from clean, unpolluted, and non-populated seas.

Dairy and dairy alternatives

Foods made from milk are valued for the protein and calcium that milk contains. For this reason, milk is recommended in varying quantities for babies, children, teens, and adults. The downsides to dairy are that the fats are saturated and it causes digestive upset for people who are lactose-intolerant.

As with fruits and vegetables, organic dairy products are better in many ways. For example, the fat content of milk from grass-fed cows is higher in omega-3 fatty acids than that of factory-farmed cows, which have almost none. Organic cows, sheep, and goats — and dairy products made from their milk — contain no drugs, growth hormones, or antibiotics.

Consider adding the following dairy products to your smoothies:

- ✔ **Cheese:** Because it's made from milk, cheese is high in protein and calcium and makes a good addition to breakfast and other meal smoothies. Soft cheeses such as cream cheese, cottage cheese, feta, and ricotta are easily added to smoothies, but you can grate firm cheeses like cheddar and Swiss before blending into smoothies, too. Be sure to check the fat content of the cheese, and make sure you don't exceed your daily calorie budget.

- ✔ **Ice cream:** Often added as a treat to fruit smoothies, ice cream is high in calories from sugar and fat. For active children and teens, ice cream milkshakes are a fun way to increase calcium in their diet, but they should be rare treats.

- ✔ **Yogurt:** This is the best dairy option — it offers calcium, protein, and cultured ("friendly") bacteria. Some lactose-sensitive people can tolerate yogurt. Probiotic yogurt helps to restore the body's natural digestive bacteria after antibiotics. Choose low-fat yogurt with "live" bacteria and use it as part of the ½ cup liquid per serving.

Vegans and lactose-intolerant people will want to look for non-dairy ingredients. Alternative cheeses, ice creams, and yogurts aren't always as high in calcium, protein, and other nutrients as those made from milk products, but their fat is unsaturated, which is a bonus.

Here are some alternatives to dairy products:

- ✔ **Rice, soy, and nut milks:** These milks are popular alternatives to animal milk. Most are fortified with vitamins A, D, B12, and calcium (check the label to be sure). Rice and almond milk have about 1 gram of protein, and soymilk has about 7 grams of protein per 8-ounce serving. Depending on the brand, rice and soymilks are available plain and in vanilla and chocolate flavors. Almond and soymilk are sweetened or not, but all varieties of rice milk are sweetened, so check the label.

- ✔ **Soy cheese:** Available in many traditional cheese varieties such as mozzarella, Parmesan, cheddar, jalapeño, and cream, soy cheeses may be available sliced, shredded, or in blocks. Soy cheese is lower in calories than its dairy counterpart, and it contains no trans fats or cholesterol. Nutrients vary by type and brand, but calcium may be added and protein is moderate, making it a popular choice for smoothies. Unlike its dairy counterpart, soy cheese has no potassium.

- ✔ **Soy ice cream:** Manufacturers of soy ice cream maintain that it contains the same ingredients used in dairy ice cream except for added oils and emulsifiers to imitate the thickness of churned cream.

  ✔ **Soy yogurt:** Made from soymilk, yogurt bacteria, and added sweeteners, soy yogurt has about the same fat as yogurt made from lower-fat milk, but it's unsaturated.

  ✔ **Tofu:** High in calcium, manganese, iron, protein, and omega-3 fats, tofu is substituted for yogurt or soy yogurt in smoothies. The silken or soft variety is best. If you get it in water-filled tubs, you can use the water as part of the liquid ingredient for smoothies.

The protein in soy is complete, meaning that it delivers all essential amino acids that the body needs for growth and repair.

Choose organic soy products because they're grown and processed in a chemical-free way.

Nuts and seeds

Studies show that eating nuts can reduce the risk of heart attacks or heart disease by 30 percent to 50 percent. In addition to their antioxidants, nuts contain the amino acid arginine, which protects the inner lining of the arterial walls, making them pliable and less susceptible to narrowing due to plaque buildup.

The Food and Drug Administration (FDA) approved this qualified health claim for nuts in 2003 by saying that science appears to point to less than two ounces of most nuts, especially almonds, if included in a whole food diet low in saturated fat and cholesterol, as being a contributing factor in reducing the risk of heart disease.

Nuts are full of fats, though, aren't they? Yes, but the fat in many nuts is healthy because it's polyunsaturated and when used in smoothies, nuts combine with the fiber to help suppress your appetite and lower your risk of weight gain. In fact, almonds, hazelnuts, pecans, walnuts, macadamia nuts, and pistachio nuts are all thought to help reduce heart disease when taken consistently. Add raw, natural, or dry-roasted nuts, and avoid nuts packaged or roasted in oil. My advice: Add 2 to 4 tablespoons of these nuts to smoothies daily. Pure natural almond butter also may be added to smoothies for heart health.

Add the following nuts to smoothies:

  ✔ **Almonds:** Lowest in calories, almonds are high in biotin and vitamin E and have a cholesterol-lowering effect due to the antioxidant action of the vitamin E. These powerhouses decrease after-meal spikes of blood sugar, which protects against diabetes and cardiovascular disease. Magnesium and potassium are important nutrients found in almonds.

✔ **Cashews:** A quarter of a cup supplies a whopping 98 percent of the daily-recommended amount of copper plus 34 percent and 33 percent of phosphorus and manganese. Copper is significant for energy and elasticity of blood vessels, bones, and joints. And cashews are lower in fat than most other nuts, almonds excluded, with about 82 percent of their fat being unsaturated and heart-healthy monounsaturated fats.

✔ **Hazelnuts:** High in vitamin A, E, and K, hazelnuts are a healthy addition to smoothies because they also add protein, complex carbohydrates, dietary fiber, iron, and calcium, while being relatively low in calories compared to other nuts.

✔ **Macadamia nuts:** High in calories (21g fat per 10 to 12 nuts), but still rich in protein, antioxidants, B-complex vitamins, and fiber, these nuts are sweet and a good addition for smoothies.

✔ **Pecans:** High in calories (20g fat per 10 to 12 nuts) but rich in monounsaturated fatty acids like oleic acid, pecans are high in antioxidants and are a good plant protein and fiber. The vitamin E and A along with lutein and zeaxanthin help protect the body from cancers and other modern diseases, like macrodegeneration.

✔ **Pistachios:** Like all nuts, pistachios are an excellent source of vitamin E, fiber, plant protein, and cholesterol-lowering mono-unsaturated fatty oils. Copper in extremely high amounts along with manganese, potassium, calcium, iron, magnesium, zinc, and selenium are also present.

✔ **Walnuts:** In addition to the heart benefits from high amounts of alpha linoleic acid, whole, natural walnuts with their skins have the added bonus of having the highest amounts of omega-3 fatty acids of any other nuts. Omega-3 fats help lower triglycerides and reduce plaque formation, and they support brain function, preventing depression and helping to increase children's attention span. About eight whole walnuts equal a 1-ounce serving.

And don't forget to add these healthful seeds to your smoothies:

✔ **Chia seeds:** They add complete protein and omega-3 fatty acids and are high in antioxidants. They're a perfect addition to smoothies because they slow the absorption of sugar into the bloodstream and bind to toxins, helping to eliminate them from the body. Soak 1 or 2 teaspoons of chia seeds in ¼ cup of juice or liquid and set aside for at least 10 minutes before adding to the liquid ingredients in smoothie recipes.

✔ **Flaxseed:** Whole flaxseeds pass through the body virtually intact without releasing their nutrients and fats, so you want to make sure to use ground flaxseed. Flaxseed contains alpha-linolenic acid (ALA), which the body uses to produce omega-3 fatty acids. Add a tablespoon of ground flaxseed to smoothies every day.

- **Hemp:** Hemp is a great vegan source of protein, fiber, and omega-6 and omega-3 fatty acids. Rich in iron, calcium, and zinc, hemp tones the skin and helps prevent anemia. Start with a teaspoon and work up to a tablespoon of hemp seeds in smoothies daily. If hemp seeds are unavailable, use wheat germ and up to a tablespoon of hemp oil.

- **Pumpkin seeds:** Although they're high in calories (559 calories per 100g), their mono-unsaturated fats help lower LDL (bad) cholesterol and increase the HDL (good) cholesterol. They're a good source of antioxidant vitamin E and the B-complex group of vitamins along with copper, manganese (almost 200 percent of the recommended-daily intake), potassium, calcium, iron, magnesium, zinc, and selenium. Regular consumption may cut the risk of prostate and ovarian cancers, so they're an excellent addition to smoothies.

- **Sunflower seeds:** Rich in the antioxidant benefits of vitamin E, sunflower seeds are perhaps the best whole food source of vitamin E, which protects against chronic diseases such as Alzheimer's and cardiovascular disease, by enhancing cell membranes, most importantly, brain cells.

Grains

I'm not pushing grains for smoothies. What do farmers feed animals to fatten them up for market? You betcha: grain, not grass. Why would human animals think they would fare any better on a high-grain diet? Here are the only grain types I *do* push:

- **Bran:** The outer and most fiber-rich part of whole grains is the *bran,* which usually gets removed from the grain during processing. It adds soluble fiber, but considerably less than psyllium. The two most popular, oat and wheat bran, contain gluten, although rice bran is available. My advice: For fiber, check out psyllium instead. (Refer to the "Super natural supplements" section later in this chapter for more information.)

- **Oatmeal:** Oatmeal is a great source of fiber that helps lower cholesterol levels and significantly reduces the risk of cardiovascular disease and stroke. The beta-glucans in oatmeal enhance the body's immune system, helping it to rid itself of fungi and bacteria. Unlike most grains, which spike blood sugar levels, oatmeal has a very low glycemic load and helps to stabilize blood sugar. With more protein than other cereal grains along with anti-inflammatory and heart-healthy antioxidants, oatmeal contains phosphorus, potassium, selenium, manganese, and iron.

✔ **Wheat germ:** The *germ* is the tiny core of the grain. It contains nutrients for the plant. Two tablespoons deliver 4 grams of protein, 2 grams of fiber, and about 1.5 grams of unsaturated fat. Hemp is richer in nutrients, but if you can tolerate gluten and don't have hemp seeds, start with a teaspoon of wheat germ and work up to a tablespoon of wheat germ in smoothies daily.

My advice: Add up to 2 tablespoons of old-fashioned, rolled oats, bran, or wheat germ per smoothie serving.

Instant oatmeal is over-processed and doesn't have the health benefits of the thicker steel-cut, old-fashioned, rolled oats.

Oats, bran, and wheat germ contain gluten, which makes them unsuitable for people who are gluten intolerant.

Herbs and spices

As a culinary herbalist, I could fill a book with the healing benefits of hundreds of herbs. Here are my top smoothie herb and spice picks:

✔ **Cinnamon:** Cinnamon can help moderate blood sugar, which is good news for diabetics and people who are weight-conscious. Cinnamon is an antioxidant and inhibits ulcers, as well as being helpful in reducing joint pain and muscle stiffness. Add ¼ teaspoon of ground cinnamon per smoothie serving.

✔ **Garlic:** Garlic's antioxidant, antibacterial, heart protecting, and anti-cancer properties give it healing power. Add one raw, peeled clove of garlic for each smoothie serving.

✔ **Ginger:** I use ginger to treat headaches, nausea, and vomiting, but ginger has anti-inflammatory and antioxidant properties, so you may want to add it to drinks often. Use 1 tablespoon of freshly grated raw ginger, ¼ teaspoon of ground ginger, or a ½-inch slice or cube of candied ginger per smoothie serving.

✔ **Licorice:** Well known as a soothing throat and stomach medicine, licorice supports the immune system. It also has anti-inflammatory and anti-tumor properties. Use ¼ to ½ teaspoon ground licorice root per smoothie serving.

✔ **Oregano:** With its powerful antioxidants and minerals — including magnesium, zinc, potassium, iron, boron, and manganese — as well as vitamins A and C, oregano is an important healing herb. Add 1 tablespoon of finely chopped fresh leaves (or 2 teaspoons dried) per serving of smoothie.

✔ **Thyme:** I grow and use thyme in cooking because of its antioxidants. Use ½ teaspoon finely chopped fresh thyme leaves per smoothie serving.

✔ **Turmeric:** The anti-inflammatory properties of turmeric help alleviate arthritis and joint pain, so add it to juices after exercising. Turmeric also fights tumors and is an antioxidant. Blend ½ teaspoon of ground turmeric per smoothie serving.

Garlic and ginger are both anticoagulants, which means that they thin the blood, so they should never be used with medications like Coumadin. If you're on blood thinners, check with your doctor before using herbs for medicinal purposes.

To read more about the healing properties of herbs, check out *Herbal Remedies For Dummies,* by Christopher Hobbs, LAc (John Wiley & Sons, Inc.) or *The Complete Guide to Medicinal Herbs,* by Penelope Ody (Dorling Kindersley).

Super natural supplements

Although chemical supplements may be convenient and promise good health, whole, natural foods offer a wide range of vitamins and minerals that are balanced with phytonutrients and in a way that complements your body. Try the following natural supplements in smoothies:

✔ **Acerola cherry:** Super high in vitamin C (32 times the amount found in orange juice) and vitamin A, acerola cherries are great. Look for them fresh or frozen or in a dried and powdered form in whole/health food stores.

✔ **Bee pollen:** Bee pollen is loaded with vitamins, amino acids, minerals, trace elements, and enzymes. Start by grinding bee pollen in a blender and then whisk 1 teaspoon per smoothie serving.

✔ **Brewer's yeast:** As a rich source of the B-complex vitamins and with essential amino acids and minerals including chromium, brewer's yeast is a good natural supplement. Add ¼ teaspoon of powder or ½ teaspoon of flakes per smoothie serving.

✔ **Dark chocolate:** Pure dark chocolate (at least 70 percent cocoa) contains flavanols and antioxidants that help prevent clogged arteries and decrease blood pressure. Pure cocoa is unsweetened and bitter, so one of the sweeteners will be required to make the drink palatable. Add 1 tablespoon of pure dark chocolate powder per smoothie serving. Add a sweetener by the teaspoon until sweetened to taste.

- **Coconut oil:** It's more solid than oil-like, but coconut oil packs a healthy punch because the fats are antimicrobial, antibacterial, and antiviral. Spoon 1 tablespoon into the blender for each smoothie serving.

- **Goji berries:** Called the longevity food, these berries are anti-inflammatory and antioxidant, which makes them important in preventing disease and the natural deterioration of cells. Goji berries are a small, dried red fruit from Asia — the best are from Tibet — that are also immune building. They're available whole dried or frozen or powdered; look for organic berries. Add up to ¼ cup to smoothie recipes.

- **Maca:** Indigenous to the Andes, maca root offers a powerful boost to the endocrine system, helps to regulate hormonal balance, and stimulates energy levels. Most often found powdered in whole/health food stores, start by adding ½ teaspoon to juice or smoothies and build up to no more than a tablespoon. Maca is not something to take every day because it can lead to adverse effects. For example, because it contains iodine, it tends to worsen the unwanted side effects of thyroid disease and may cause goiters. It may also promote allergic symptoms like hives, fatigue, and rash that may develop with prolonged use. For these reasons, you should consider consulting your healthcare provider before taking maca.

- **Psyllium:** Psyllium is the outer husk or covering of the plant known as *Plantago ovata*. Its soluble fiber absorbs water, forms a gel, and swells, putting pressure on the colon and easing constipation. Add a teaspoon to a smoothie serving, and drink a glass of water after the smoothie and several glasses of water throughout the day.

- **Propolis:** Bees mix a resinous sap from trees with wax and use it for general hive maintenance; this sap is called *propolis*. With its ability to fight infection and its antimicrobial, antioxidant, anti-ulcer, and antitumor qualities, propolis is great for humans, too. Add 2 teaspoons per smoothie serving.

- **Reishi mushroom:** A tree mushroom, it increases immunity and is antiviral. It's often included in tonics and may help reduce stress by calming the mind while strengthening the brain and nervous system and normalizing body processes. It may be available in powdered form, but you can purchase it in gel capsules; empty 2 and add to the smoothie or juice ingredients. Use about 1 teaspoon or 2 capsules.

- **Umeboshi:** A paste made from pickled plums, this Asian health food is valued for its antibacterial and pH balancing effect. Best of all, it's used to curb sugar addiction and cravings. Add 1 teaspoon per smoothie serving.

> ✔ **Whey protein powder:** Protein builds cells, muscle, bones, neurotransmitters, hormones, and antibodies, and it assists metabolism, making it helpful to weight loss. Whey protein does all this and it stimulates the immune system. Choose whey protein isolate over whey protein concentrate (because it contains less lactose and more protein) and scoop 2 to 4 tablespoons into the blender for smoothies.

Tinctures, tonic teas, and elixirs

Tinctures are concentrated extractions of the active components of plants that have been dissolved in alcohol. *Tonics* and *elixirs* are herbal drinks that are made from tonic herbs and may use tinctures, or they may be simple teas or even smoothies. It is their effect on the body that makes them tonic. All offer a convenient way to add the benefits of medicinal herbs to your daily routine.

The Herbal Home Remedy Book: Simple Recipes for Tinctures, Teas, Salves, Tonics and Syrups, by Joyce A. Wardwell (Storey Publishing), offers more information on this topic.

Tinctures

The whole or specific parts of an herb are immersed in alcohol to extract their active components. Tinctures are available in whole-food or health food stores. Some tincture herbs are astragalus and echinacea for immune boosting; valerian and hops to calm nerves; dandelion and milk thistle to cleanse; and ginseng and mint to refresh and stimulate. You can add tinctures by the drop to juices. Follow guidelines for doses given by the manufacturer or a qualified herbalist.

Tonic teas

Tonic herbs are considered superior because they strengthen the body and prevent illness (as opposed to medicinal or inferior herbs, which treat illness). Tonic herbs such as parsley, basil, and stinging nettles balance and nourish; ginseng, astragalus, and licorice help the body to adjust to stress, aging, and pollutants.

Elixirs

Teas or whole herb liquid extractions made from tonic herbs often are combined with natural, healthy supplements. These drinks are called elixirs. Juices made with antioxidant fruits and/or vegetables that also include a tonic tea or tincture are great-tasting elixirs.

Sweeteners

Only four sweeteners can be considered healthy:

- ✔ **Stevia:** Stevia is an herb with leaves that are up to 300 times sweeter, gram for gram, than sugar. The most exciting thing about stevia is that it has no effect on blood glucose, so you get the sweet taste without the high blood sugar boom and bust. Stevia is available in dried whole or cut-leaf form, powder, and syrup or extract. The extract is easiest to use in smoothies, but I've used the powder, too. Start with a small amount and taste before adding more.

- ✔ **Blackstrap molasses:** When cane sugar is processed or boiled into refined, white sugar, one of the by-products is mineral-rich, thick, and tart-tasting molasses. Blackstrap molasses results from the last of the boiling of the cane sugar. It is lower in sugar than any of the other molasses types. It's a good source of potassium, copper, iron, calcium, manganese, and magnesium, so add 1 tablespoon to each smoothie serving.

- ✔ **Coconut nectar:** It's a sweet, syrupy sweetener that is a product of the sap from coconut trees. With only around 10 percent fructose, it's low glycemic and contains some active enzymes and minerals. Add it to taste to smoothies and vegetable juices.

- ✔ **Raw, unfiltered honey:** Many of honey's phytonutrients and enzymes are destroyed by pasteurization and high heat processing, so raw (unpasteurized) honey is ideal. Unfortunately, it's almost impossible to find unless you have a beehive in your backyard. Also, the harder the honey, the higher the nutrients, but the more difficult it is to incorporate into drinks. My advice: Choose blackstrap molasses or stevia over honey if all you can get is the pasteurized, liquid honey in a cute bear-shaped jar.

Making Smoothies: Some Easy Techniques to Follow

Smoothies are super-easy to make, so there isn't a whole lot to master in the way of technique. But in this section I give you some pointers that make incorporating smoothies into your daily life even easier.

Peeling, seeding, coring, and chopping

All fruits and vegetables — organic or not — should be washed with either food-safe soap and water or vinegar and water. This, along with proper storage, (see Chapter 4) is the first step in keeping produce fresh and safe, and it's worth repeating.

All inedible skin, rind, or peel on fruits and vegetables must be removed and discarded before blending. If the produce is organic, the nutrient-rich skin should be left on (if it's not organic, you should peel the skin). You don't need to remove the edible seeds from the following fruits and vegetables:

- ✔ Blackberry
- ✔ Blueberry
- ✔ Cucumber
- ✔ Eggplant
- ✔ Kiwifruit
- ✔ Okra
- ✔ Papaya
- ✔ Pomegranate
- ✔ Raspberry
- ✔ Snap beans and pods
- ✔ Squash
- ✔ Star fruit
- ✔ Strawberry
- ✔ Tomato
- ✔ Watermelon (from "seedless" varieties)

The core (not the seeds) of pears and apples, while normally too tough to eat, may be left on the fruit if the blender is powerful enough to cut them into fine, drinkable particles.

The seeds of apples, apricots, peaches, pears, and plums contain tiny amounts of cyanide compounds and should be discarded before juicing or blending.

Here's how to prepare a variety of fruits and vegetables for the blender:

- ✔ **Apples:** Cut into eighths; leave the skin on if organic; deseed.
- ✔ **Apricots:** Halve; leave the skin on if organic; remove the stones.
- ✔ **Banana:** Peel and cut into four pieces.

- **Beans:** Leave whole; halve large.
- **Beets:** Cut into 1-inch pieces; leave the skin on if organic.
- **Berries:** Leave whole; halve large.
- **Carrots:** Cut into 1-inch pieces; leave the skin on if organic.
- **Citrus fruits:** Peel and quarter; deseed.
- **Cucumber:** Peel and cut into four pieces. Leave the skin on if organic.
- **Garlic cloves:** Leave whole; halve large.
- **Kiwifruit:** Peel and quarter.
- **Mango:** Peel and quarter, cut stone out.
- **Nectarine:** Halve; leave the skin on if organic; remove the stones.
- **Onions:** Peel and cut into eighths.
- **Papaya:** Peel and quarter.
- **Peaches:** Halve; leave the skin on if organic; remove the stones.
- **Peas:** Leave whole.
- **Plums:** Halve; leave the skin on if organic; remove the stones.
- **Pumpkins:** Cut into 1-inch pieces; remove skin and seeds.
- **Squash:** Cut into 1-inch pieces; remove skin and seeds.
- **Starfruit:** Peel and quarter.
- **Strawberries:** Leave whole; halve large.
- **Summer squash:** Peel and cut into four pieces if small. Leave the skin on if organic.
- **Tomato:** Quarter; leave the skin on if organic.

Doing things in order

Always add liquid to the container of the blender first, because it allows the blades to spin unencumbered until the chunks of food get drawn down, cut, and then liquefied. The recipes in this book tell you what order to add ingredients to the blender.

Blending frozen ingredients

If your blender has a pulse button feature and it's made to handle ice, follow these steps to blend frozen ingredients (for one serving):

1. **Pour ½ cup liquid into the container.**

2. **Add 2 cups of frozen fruits, vegetables, or ice.**

3. **Place the lid on the container and pulse the blender five or six times in quick, two-second bursts.**

4. **Push the Chop or Crush button and process for 15 to 30 seconds.**

   If the ice gets stuck, stop the blender and use a spatula or the handle of a wooden spoon to move the smaller pieces out of the way of the blades and pulse again. If you don't have a Chop or Crush button, keep pulsing for another five or six times and then proceed to Steps 5 and 6.

5. **With the motor running, you can add up to 1 cup of unfrozen ingredients through the opening in the lid.**

   Only fill the container up to three-fourths full.

6. **Process on high for 30 to 40 seconds or until the smoothie is the consistency you want.**

If you only want to crush ice for drinks, don't add water as directed in Step 1 and stop the blender after Step 4. If you have a stir stick, use it to stir up larger chunks and get them moving toward the blades while the motor is running. If not, stop and use a wooden spoon as directed in Step 4.

The easiest way to crush ice without using a blender is to fill a resealable plastic bag with ice so that, when sealed and laying flat, the bag has only one layer of cubes. Use a hammer or rolling pin to smash the ice into small pieces. You can add these smaller pieces to smoothie ingredients in the blender to make a thick and frozen drink.

Chapter 16

Crafting Some Tasty Fruit Smoothies

Drinking fruit at breakfast and for early morning snacks gives you energy in the form of *natural* fructose (fruit sugar). The difference between juices and smoothies is that juicing requires many more individual fruits and juicing separates out the fiber, so the nutrients and the natural fruit sugars are concentrated. On the other hand, smoothies are made from one or two whole fruits, which means that the fruit sugars are bound up in the fiber or carbohydrate cellulose of the fruit and released into the bloodstream slowly. This keeps blood sugar levels even, and that, in turn, means that mood swings and spikes in energy don't occur.

The natural sweetness from fruit smoothies is far superior to fast-food snacks, which are full of refined sugars that spike and then leave you feeling slightly deflated and craving more. This natural sweetness makes them delicious breakfasts, snacks, and alcoholic and nonalcoholic drinks. Even better, they can be used as desserts.

This chapter focuses specifically on different smoothies that you can try. If you want some dessert smoothie recipes, check out www.dummies.com/extras/juicingsmoothies for a few.

Breakfast and Snack Fruit Smoothies

Smoothies have some advantages over juices. First, they're very easy to prepare, so you can make fruit smoothies in the morning without having to precut the ingredients. If you have flaxseed or hemp and other healthy smoothie ingredients ready to measure out, the job of creating a delicious, portable breakfast or snack is fast and convenient. If you have a portable, one-serving blending machine, you can measure out all the ingredients you need for one or two snacks, pack them in a cooler, and make satisfying smoothies for a health break at work.

The second benefit of smoothies is that cleanup is simple. The machine actually does the work in cleaning the blades and the container in seconds, so you can have the drink made, the machine cleaned up, and be out the door or back to work in minutes.

Here are some ingredients to add at breakfast and snack time:

- ✓ **Oatmeal:** Large flake (rolled oats, old-fashioned oatmeal, not instant); 2 tablespoons per serving.

- ✓ **Nuts:** Chopped almonds, hazelnuts, pecans, walnuts, macadamia nuts, or pistachio nuts; 2 to 4 tablespoons.

- ✓ **Yogurt and low-fat milk:** Use milk as the liquid and add ¼ cup yogurt per serving.

- ✓ **Cheese:** Soft cheeses like feta, goat cheese, or medium cheese such as cheddar, Havarti, or Swiss for calcium and protein; 1 to 2 tablespoons or 1-inch cubes per serving.

- ✓ **Tofu:** For calcium, manganese, iron, protein, and omega-3 fatty acids; ¼ cup silken or soft tofu per serving.

- ✓ **Flaxseed:** Use ground flaxseeds to add omega-3 fatty acids; 1 tablespoon ground flaxseeds per serving daily.

If you suffer from poor digestion, be mindful of combining protein ingredients — like yogurt, cottage cheese, nuts, or seeds — with fruit in smoothies. The body sends different enzymes to the gut for digesting proteins and, in some people, fruit prevents those enzymes from doing their job. Some fruits have natural digestive agents that can be combined in a smoothie to help remedy this problem. Chapter 12 offers some tips on natural digestive ingredients you can add to smoothies.

Banana Breakfast

Prep time: About 3 min • **Blending time:** 1 min • **Yield:** 2 servings

Ingredients	Directions
2 ripe bananas	**1** Peel the bananas and break each into 4 chunks.
½ cup low-fat milk	
1 cup fresh or frozen blueberries	**2** Combine the milk, bananas, blueberries, flaxseed, and yogurt in the blender container.
1 tablespoon ground flaxseed	**3** Secure the lid on the container.
⅔ cup plain, low-fat yogurt	**4** Starting on a low speed and gradually easing toward high, blend the ingredients for 45 seconds or until smooth and there are no visible pieces of fruit in the mixture.
	5 Pour the smoothie into 2 glasses and enjoy!

Per serving: Calories 247 (From Fat 37); Fat 4g (Saturated 2g); Cholesterol 7mg; Sodium 96mg; Carbohydrate 48g (Dietary Fiber 6g); Protein 9g.

Vary It! Bananas are a great source of potassium, which is thought to play a role in controlling high blood pressure, but some people just don't like them. If you fall into the anti-banana camp, you can substitute any one of the following for the bananas: one sliced avocado; ⅓ cup old-fashioned rolled oats (large-flake oatmeal); ⅓ cup silken tofu; or 2 tablespoons chia seeds soaked for ten minutes in the milk plus two peeled and pitted mangoes.

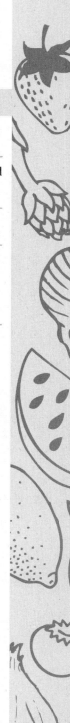

Get Up and Go

Prep time: About 4 min • **Blending time:** 1 min • **Yield:** 2 servings

Ingredients	Directions
2 mangoes	*1* Peel the mangoes, cut them in half, and remove the flat stone from each.
1 orange	
¾ cup freshly squeezed orange juice	*2* Peel the orange and break it into segments. Remove the seeds.
1 cup frozen fruit chunks	
½ cup low-fat cottage cheese	*3* Combine the orange juice, mangoes, orange, frozen fruit, and cheese in the blender container.
	4 Secure the lid on the container.
	5 Starting on a low speed and gradually easing toward high, blend the ingredients for 45 seconds or until smooth and there are no visible pieces of fruit in the mixture.
	6 Pour the smoothie into 2 glasses and enjoy!

Per serving: Calories 287 (From Fat 16); Fat 2g (Saturated 1g); Cholesterol 2mg; Sodium 236mg; Carbohydrate 64g (Dietary Fiber 7g); Protein 10g.

Tip: You can use mixed, commercially frozen berries or fruit chunks, or you can slice and freeze any fruit that is in season, including tree fruit, stone fruit, and berries for this recipe. This smoothie is very thick! If you prefer a thinner version, add more orange juice: ¼ to ½ cup extra for a slightly thinner smoothie, or 1 cup extra for a very thin smoothie.

Berry Nutty

Prep time: About 2 min • **Blending time:** 1 min • **Yield:** 2 servings

Ingredients	Directions
⅓ cup cranberry juice	**1** Combine the cranberry juice, pomegranate juice, blueberries or blackberries, acai berries, tofu, and walnuts in the blender container.
¼ cup pomegranate juice	
1 cup fresh blueberries or blackberries	**2** Secure the lid on the container.
1 cup frozen acai berries	**3** Starting on a low speed and gradually easing toward high, blend the ingredients for 45 seconds or until smooth and there are no visible pieces of fruit or nuts in the mixture.
⅓ cup silken tofu	
2 tablespoons chopped walnuts	
	4 Pour the smoothie into 2 glasses and enjoy!

Per serving: Calories 203 (From Fat 78); Fat 9g (Saturated 1g); Cholesterol 0mg; Sodium 10mg; Carbohydrate 29g (Dietary Fiber 4g); Protein 4g.

Vary It! You can use plain low-fat yogurt in place of the tofu.

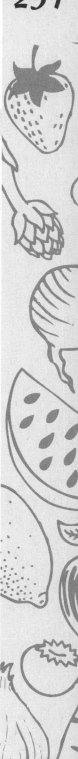

Tropical Pick-Me-Up

Prep time: About 2 min • **Blending time:** 1 min • **Yield:** 2 servings

Ingredients	Directions
1 cup coconut cream or coconut milk	**1** Combine the coconut cream or milk and whey powder and blend for a few seconds to combine.
2 tablespoons whey protein powder	
1 cup cantaloupe melon pieces	**2** Peel the banana and break it into 4 chunks. Add banana chunks, melon, peaches, and Brazil nuts (if using) in the blender container.
1 cup frozen peach slices	
1 banana	**3** Secure the lid on the container.
1 tablespoon chopped Brazil nuts (optional)	**4** Starting on a low speed and gradually easing toward high, blend the ingredients for 45 seconds or until smooth and there are no visible pieces of fruit or nuts in the mixture.
	5 Pour the smoothie into 2 glasses and enjoy!

Per serving: Calories 472 (From Fat 271); Fat 30g (Saturated 25g); Cholesterol 0mg; Sodium 144mg; Carbohydrate 46g (Dietary Fiber 8g); Protein 12g.

Vary It! You can substitute pineapple for the peaches. You also can add toasted coconut shreds as a garnish.

Tip: Coconut cream is a thick, pastelike liquid that is pressed from the coconut flesh, so it's similar to and yet thicker than coconut milk. You can make your own coconut cream by blending fresh coconut flesh with a small amount of water.

Adding Healthy Ingredients

I'm convinced that the human diet determines to a great extent, a person's health. It only makes sense that if your cells, tissue, bones, muscles and organs have life-giving, strengthening nutrients and specific enzymes for optimum functioning and preventing disease, then you'll be strong and resist disease. You're already giving your body a powerful gift by juicing and making smoothies, so why not go the distance and discover more about the kinds of healthy ingredients you can add for specific body functions?

Adrenal and endocrine smoothie elixirs

Your adrenal glands (located on top of your kidneys) are important because they run the show or call the shots, so to speak. By secreting hormones (including cortisol) that trigger certain functions in different body tissues, the adrenal glands produce chemical messengers, which regulate metabolism, blood pressure, and direct your involuntary response to stress. Keeping the adrenal glands working at optimum means that you can avoid suffering from fatigue, which can be seriously debilitating.

Like your adrenal glands, your endocrine glands also secrete hormones into the bloodstream, which regulate several functions, including growth, reproduction, energy, bone and muscle strength, and metabolism. The endocrine glands include hypothalamus, pineal, pituitary, thyroid, parathyroid, thymus, adrenal, pancreas, ovaries, and testes. As one of your body's important communication systems, hormone imbalances can result in hypo- or hyperglycemia (high or low blood sugar), hypo- or hyperthyroidism (slow or fast thyroid/metabolic function), among other symptoms.

The smoothie recipes in this section can help keep your adrenal and endocrine glands operating smoothly.

Mighty Maca

Prep time: About 2 min • **Blending time:** 1 min • **Yield:** 2 servings

Ingredients	Directions
1 mango or 1 cup chopped frozen mango	*1* Peel and stone the mango and chop the flesh.
1 cup almond or coconut milk	*2* Combine the almond milk, mango, frozen berries, banana, and maca powder in the blender container.
1 cup frozen berries	
1 fresh or frozen banana	*3* Secure the lid on the container.
2 teaspoons powdered maca powder	*4* Starting on a low speed and gradually easing toward high, pulse the ingredients for 30 seconds. Check the consistency and blend on high for 10 to 20 seconds or until smooth.
	5 Pour the smoothie into 2 glasses and enjoy!

Per serving: Calories 195 (From Fat 23); Fat 3g (Saturated 0g); Cholesterol 0mg; Sodium 74mg; Carbohydrate 45g (Dietary Fiber 5g); Protein 2g.

Tip: Try to balance the fresh and frozen mangoes or berries in this recipe because if both are frozen, the result will be a very thick smoothie.

Reishi Rush

Prep time: About 1 min • **Blending time:** 1 min • **Yield:** 1 serving

Ingredients	Directions
1 cup almond or coconut milk	*1* Combine the almond or coconut milk, powdered cacao, nectar or honey, and banana in the blender container.
1 tablespoon powdered, non-sweetened dark chocolate cacao	
1 tablespoon coconut nectar or honey	*2* Open the capsules and pour reishi powder and maca over the ingredients in the blender container.
1 fresh or frozen banana	*3* Secure the lid on the container.
2 reishi capsules	*4* Starting on a low speed and gradually easing toward high, blend the ingredients for 30 seconds or until smooth.
½ teaspoon maca powder	
	5 Pour the smoothie into 2 glasses and enjoy!

Per serving: Calories 211 (From Fat 48); Fat 5g (Saturated 2g); Cholesterol 0mg; Sodium 153mg; Carbohydrate 40g (Dietary Fiber 6g); Protein 4g.

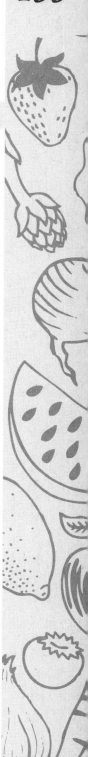

Antioxidant smoothies

Brightly colored fruits and vegetables (blueberries, acai berries, goji berries, red peppers), bright green leafy vegetables (spinach, kale, Swiss chard), and other ingredients (dark chocolate, chia seeds, and red wine) have the ability to complete the missing parts of damaging free radicals, thus rendering them harmless to the body's cells. Some of the same ingredients are anti-inflammatory, making them doubly important in disease prevention.

In the following recipes, I include some of the following anti-aging, anti-disease, anti-oxidant ingredients in smoothies. Try them and see how easy it is to punch up the already high antioxidant power of bright fruit and vegetables by adding other ingredients, such as the following:

- Chia seeds
- Goji berries
- Dark chocolate (79 percent cacao or more)
- Black and green tea
- Green herbs, such as thyme, oregano, rosemary, and sage

Chia Bowl

Prep time: About 12 min • **Blending time:** 1 min • **Yield:** 2 servings

Ingredients	Directions
½ cup almond or coconut milk	**1** Combine the almond milk and chia seeds in the blender container. Set aside for 10 minutes to thicken.
¼ cup chia seeds	
¼ cup apple juice	**2** Add the apple juice, blueberries, and kale (see Figure 16-1) to the soaked chia seeds in the blender container. Secure the lid on the container.
1 cup fresh or frozen blueberries	
1 cup fresh or frozen kale	**3** Starting on a low speed and gradually easing toward high, pulse the ingredients for 30 seconds. Check the consistency and blend on high for 10 to 20 seconds or until smooth. Add more apple juice to thin the drink if necessary.
	4 Pour the smoothie into 2 glasses and enjoy!

Per serving: Calories 190 (From Fat 69); Fat 8g (Saturated 1g); Cholesterol 0mg; Sodium 54mg; Carbohydrate 28g (Dietary Fiber 10g); Protein 6g.

Tip: You can add another ¼ cup almond or coconut milk to thin this smoothie.

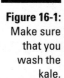

Figure 16-1: Make sure that you wash the kale.

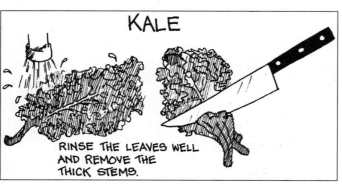

Illustration by Elizabeth Kurtzman

Go-To Goji

Prep time: About 12 min • **Blending time:** 1 min • **Yield:** 2 servings

Ingredients	Directions
¾ cup fresh orange or carrot juice 1 cup fresh or frozen (thawed) pomegranate seeds or raspberries ½ cup fresh or frozen (thawed) strawberries ¼ cup dried or frozen goji berries	**1** Combine the orange or carrot juice, pomegranate seeds or raspberries, strawberries, and goji berries in the blender container. Set aside for 10 minutes to plump and soften the goji berries.
	2 Secure the lid on the container.
	3 Starting on a low speed and gradually easing toward high, pulse the ingredients for 30 seconds. Check the consistency and blend on high for 10 to 20 seconds or until smooth.
	4 Pour the smoothie into 2 glasses and enjoy!

Per serving: Calories 179 (From Fat 12); Fat 1g (Saturated 0g); Cholesterol 0mg; Sodium 54mg; Carbohydrate 40g (Dietary Fiber 5g); Protein 4g.

Enjoying Exercise and Energy Smoothies

You can definitely fuel and restore spent glycogen from your workout with the natural fructose in plant carbohydrates (sugars and starches), but you likely already know this. Because they're quick, easy to digest, and can include so many nutritious ingredients, smoothies are the perfect snack to include in your exercise routine. Drink them immediately following your activity for maximum support in restoring energy and repairing muscle tissue.

Want to push the envelope? Start with the following recipes and try adding the following energy-building and exercise-supporting ingredients to your favorite smoothies.

✔ A banana provides potassium.

✔ Nuts like pecans, walnuts, and almonds provide protein for muscles and increase healthy fats for energy.

✔ Turmeric helps ease post-exercise pain.

✔ Avocados contain cholesterol-lowering fats, which improve cardio health.

✔ Kale and other green leafy vegetables are rich in vitamins A, C, and K, with calcium and iron for improving bone and muscle performance.

✔ Extra virgin coconut oil or olive oil provide essential fatty acids and energy for moving bodies.

Hemp Help

Prep time: About 2 min   •   **Blending time:** 1 min   •   **Yield:** 1 to 2 servings

Ingredients	Directions
1 orange	**1** Peel the orange, leaving the white pith. Separate into sections and seed if necessary.
1 cup almond or coconut milk	
2 tablespoons unsalted cashews	**2** Combine the almond or coconut milk, cashews, coconut oil, hemp hearts, orange sections, and berries in the blender container.
1 tablespoon coconut oil	
¼ cup hemp hearts or seeds	**3** Secure the lid on the container.
1 cup fresh or frozen berries	**4** Starting on a low speed and gradually easing toward high, pulse the ingredients for 30 seconds. Check the consistency and blend on high for 10 to 20 seconds or until smooth.
	5 Pour the smoothie into 2 glasses and enjoy!

Per serving: Calories 318 (From Fat 178); Fat 20g (Saturated 7g); Cholesterol 0mg; Sodium 75mg; Carbohydrate 27g (Dietary Fiber 6g); Protein 10g.

Mango-Turmeric Cool-Down

Prep time: About 2 min • **Blending time:** 1 min • **Yield:** 2 servings

Ingredients	Directions
2 mangoes	*1* Peel and stone the mangoes and coarsely chop the flesh.
1 cup carrot or orange juice	
1 tablespoon coconut oil	*2* Combine the carrot or orange juice, coconut oil, mangoes, banana, turmeric, and ginger in the blender container.
1 fresh or frozen banana	
¼ teaspoon powdered turmeric	*3* Secure the lid on the container.
¼ teaspoon chopped fresh or powdered ginger	*4* Starting on a low speed and gradually easing toward high, pulse the ingredients for 30 seconds. Check the consistency and blend on high for 10 to 20 seconds or until smooth.
	5 Pour the smoothie into 2 glasses and enjoy!

Per serving: Calories 309 (From Fat 72); Fat 8g (Saturated 6g); Cholesterol 0mg; Sodium 0mg; Carbohydrate 61g (Dietary Fiber 4g); Protein 2g.

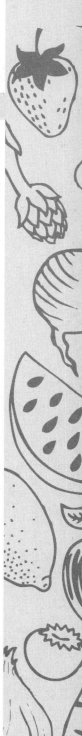

The Bees' Best

Prep time: About 2 min • **Blending time:** 1 min • **Yield:** 2 servings

Ingredients	Directions
2 papayas	**1** Peel the papayas, leaving seeds intact and coarsely chop the flesh. Peel the banana and cut into 4 to 6 chunks.
1 fresh or frozen banana	
1 cup almond or coconut milk	**2** Combine the almond or coconut milk, honey or coconut nectar, papayas, banana, and pollen in the blender container.
1 tablespoon honey or coconut nectar	
1 teaspoon bee pollen	**3** Secure the lid on the container.
	4 Starting on a low speed and gradually easing toward high, pulse the ingredients for 30 seconds. Check the consistency and blend on high for 10 to 20 seconds or until smooth.
	5 Pour the smoothie into 2 glasses and enjoy!

Per serving: Calories 189 (From Fat 18); Fat 2g (Saturated 0g); Cholesterol 0mg; Sodium 87mg; Carbohydrate 44g (Dietary Fiber 5g); Protein 3g.

Tip: If this smoothie is too thick for you, add more milk until it is exactly the way you like it.

Focusing on Immunity-Building Smoothies

Like the immune-boosting juices in Chapter 12, smoothies can also take advantage of the same natural, antioxidant ingredients. Antioxidants are essential to boosting immunity because they help to keep your body's tissues in good repair so that they can resist disease. Use at least one of the following antioxidant fruits in smoothies for immunity:

- **Black or blue fruit:** Plums, blue/black berries, red or black cherries, acai berries, gooseberries
- **Bright red fruit or vegetables:** Raspberries, pomegranate seeds, strawberries, red bell peppers
- **Bright green fruit or vegetables:** Broccoli, kale, spinach, Swiss chard, herbs (rosemary, sage, thyme)

These recipes introduce some relatively new antioxidant ingredients. All are available in powder form from natural/health food stores.

- Acerola cherries are rich in Vitamin C (32 times the amount found in orange juice) and vitamin A for antioxidant punch.
- Kombucha, often called *kombucha tea,* is a fermented drink made from tea, sugar, bacteria, and yeast that is often found in grocery stores. Although many of its health claims are as yet unproven, like other fermented foods, it may serve to strengthen the immune system. You may substitute it with soft apple cider in the recipe in this section.
- Macha tea is finely powdered green tea that adds an earthy, grassy taste along with about 23 times the antioxidant power of acai berries.
- Moringa leaves are dried and added to smoothies because of their protein, potassium, and calcium as well as their high antioxidant components.

Great Green Smoothie

Prep time: About 2 min • **Blending time:** 1 min • **Yield:** 2 servings

Ingredients	Directions
2 black plums	**1** Cut the plums in half and remove the stones.
½ avocado	**2** Peel, seed, and chop the avocado half.
¾ cup white grape juice	**3** Combine the grape juice, lime juice, cherry powder, pomegranate seeds, kale or spinach, plums, and avocado (see Figure 16-2) in the blender container.
¼ cup freshly squeezed lime juice	
1 teaspoon acerola cherry powder	
1 cup fresh or frozen pomegranate seeds	**4** Secure the lid on the container.
1 cup coarsely chopped kale or spinach	**5** Starting on a low speed and gradually easing toward high, pulse the ingredients for 30 seconds. Check the consistency and blend on high for 10 to 20 seconds or until smooth.
	6 Pour the smoothie into 2 glasses and enjoy!

Per serving: Calories 251 (From Fat 64); Fat 7g (Saturated 1g); Cholesterol 0mg; Sodium 22mg; Carbohydrate 48g (Dietary Fiber 6g); Protein 5g.

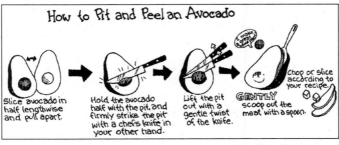

Figure 16-2: Pitting and peeling an avocado.

How to Pit and Peel an Avocado

Slice avocado in half lengthwise and pull apart.

Hold the avocado half with the pit, and firmly strike the pit with a chef's knife in your other hand.

Lift the pit out with a gentle twist of the knife.

GENTLY scoop out the meat with a spoon.

chop or slice according to your recipe.

Illustration by Elizabeth Kurtzman

Kombucha

Prep time: About 2 min • **Blending time:** 1 min • **Yield:** 2 servings

Ingredients	Directions
½ cup kombucha 1 tablespoon coconut oil 2 tablespoons coconut nectar or liquid honey 1 cup fresh or frozen blueberries 1 cup fresh or frozen strawberries 1 cup coarsely chopped spinach	*1* Combine the kombucha, coconut oil, coconut nectar or honey, blueberries, strawberries, and spinach in the blender container. *2* Secure the lid on the container. *3* Starting on a low speed and gradually easing toward high, pulse the ingredients for 30 seconds. Check the consistency and blend on high for 10 to 20 seconds or until smooth. *4* Pour the smoothie into 2 glasses and enjoy!

Per serving: Calories 205 (From Fat 63); Fat 7g (Saturated 6g); Cholesterol 0mg; Sodium 22mg; Carbohydrate 38g (Dietary Fiber 4g); Protein 2g.

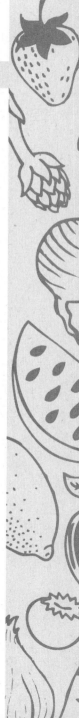

Purple Punch

Prep time: About 2 min • **Blending time:** 1 min • **Yield:** 2 servings

Ingredients	Directions
1 cup pomegranate juice	**1** Combine the pomegranate juice, cherry powder, cherries, blueberries, and kale or spinach in the blender container.
1 teaspoon acerola cherry powder	
1 cup fresh or frozen black cherries	**2** Secure the lid on the container.
1 cup fresh or frozen blueberries	**3** Starting on a low speed and gradually easing toward high, pulse the ingredients for 30 seconds. Check the consistency and blend on high for 10 to 20 seconds or until smooth.
1 cup coarsely chopped kale or spinach	
	4 Pour the smoothie into 2 glasses and enjoy!

Per serving: Calories 179 (From Fat 5); Fat 1g (Saturated 0g); Cholesterol 0mg; Sodium 29mg; Carbohydrate 44g (Dietary Fiber 4g); Protein 3g.

Making Fruit Mocktail and Cocktail Smoothies

If you enjoy getting together for the occasional end-of-the-week drink with friends, you can pick up some ideas in this section about how to choose nourishing beverages that can work within an overall healthy diet.

Fruit mocktails are festive, social smoothies without alcohol. Because they tend to be high in calories, they're best consumed as an occasional treat. The fruit sugars make them hard to resist, and they're so delicious that I'd wager even people who actually drink alcohol would make the switch, but designated drivers, pregnant women, or anyone choosing not to consume alcohol will thank you for making them. You can make up a blender full half an hour before an event, pour them into shot glasses, and freeze them — just leave about ¾ inch headspace at the top of the smoothies and take them out of the freezer within a couple hours so they don't freeze rock solid.

 Fruit smoothie cocktails are really just the same delicious smoothies as mocktails with 1 ounce of alcohol per serving added to the liquids. You can turn any of the fruit smoothies in this chapter into a cocktail worthy of the best mixologist. *Note:* For each ounce of alcohol spirits you add to a drink, you're adding about 100 calories.

Rimming mocktail and cocktail glasses

Rimming glasses is fun and easy to do. All you need is 1 cup granulated sugar, 1 tablespoon of your favorite ground spice (like cinnamon) or freshly chopped herb (such as mint), and 1 or 2 lime or lemon wedges. Follow these steps:

1. **In a small bowl, combine the sugar and the spice or herb.**

2. **Spread the mixture evenly into a saucer or shallow bowl.**

3. **Use a lime or lemon wedge to run around and wet the rim of each glass.**

4. **Turn the glasses upside down and set the moistened rims into the sugar mixture.**

5. **Twist and lift out.**

Use a rimming mixture for one evening or event and then discard it. Bacteria can grow in the mixture after it's moistened.

Strawberry Daiquiri Decoy

Prep time: About 3 min • **Blending time:** 1 min • **Yield:** 2 servings

Ingredients	Directions
½ cup cranberry or pomegranate juice	**1** Combine the cranberry or pomegranate juice, lime juice, and strawberries in the blender container.
3 tablespoons fresh lime juice	**2** Secure the lid on the container.
¾ cup frozen strawberries	**3** Starting on a low speed and gradually easing toward high, blend the ingredients for 30 seconds. Add ice and pulse for 20 seconds or until ice is evenly mixed in.
¼ cup crushed ice	**4** Pour the smoothie into 2 glasses and enjoy!

Per serving: Calories 59 (From Fat 3); Fat 0 (Saturated 0g); Cholesterol 0mg; Sodium 2mg; Carbohydrate 15g (Dietary Fiber 2g); Protein 0g.

Tip: Add more lime juice until the desired sourness is achieved.

Don't speed

The key to preserving your blender and making great smoothies is to start at a low speed in order to get the blades moving, and then turn up the speed to medium and watch as the larger chunks of ingredients begin to break up. When the pieces of fruits and vegetables are liquidizing and being forced up and around the sides of the container, ease the dial up toward High. If you increase the speed too quickly, a large air bubble will form, and the blades will just spin around inside it.

Nada Piña Colada

Prep time: About 3 min • **Blending time:** 1 min • **Yield:** 2 servings

Ingredients	Directions
½ cup pineapple juice	**1** Combine the pineapple juice, coconut cream or milk, and pineapple chunks in the blender container.
¼ cup coconut cream or coconut milk	
¾ cup frozen pineapple chunks	**2** Secure the lid on the container.
¼ cup crushed ice	**3** Starting on a low speed and gradually easing toward high, blend the ingredients for 30 seconds. Add ice and pulse for 20 seconds or until ice is evenly mixed in.
	4 Pour the smoothie into 2 glasses and enjoy!

Per serving: Calories 135 (From Fat 62); Fat 7g (Saturated 6g); Cholesterol 0mg; Sodium 20mg; Carbohydrate 19g (Dietary Fiber 2g); Protein 1g.

Tip: Coconut cream is a thick, pastelike liquid that is pressed from the coconut flesh, so it's similar to and yet thicker than coconut milk. You can make your own coconut cream by blending fresh coconut flesh with a small amount of water.

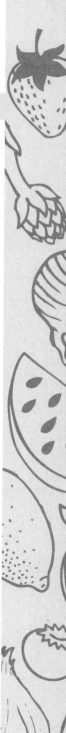

Peach Mixer

Prep time: About 3 min • **Blending time:** 1 min • **Yield:** 2 servings

Ingredients	Directions
½ cup peach or apricot nectar	**1** Combine the nectar, lemon juice, alcohol, and peaches in the blender container.
2 tablespoons fresh lemon juice	
2 ounces rum, gin, or vodka	**2** Secure the lid on the container.
¾ cup frozen peach slices	**3** Starting on a low speed and gradually easing toward high, blend the ingredients for 30 seconds. Add ice and pulse for 20 seconds or until ice is evenly mixed in.
¼ cup crushed ice	**4** Pour the smoothie into 2 glasses and enjoy!

Per serving: Calories 130 (From Fat 0); Fat 0g (Saturated 0g); Cholesterol 0mg; Sodium 5mg; Carbohydrate 17g (Dietary Fiber 2g); Protein 1g.

Vary It! You can use pineapple or apple juice in place of the nectar. Peaches, nectarines, plums, and apricots may be sliced, frozen, and substituted in this recipe.

Preparing fruit

If you really want to get everything ready for a smoothie in advance, try these tips:

- Buy organic ingredients so that you don't have to peel them.

- Wash fruit and vegetables the night before, but leave them whole unless they take a long time to cut up.

- Store peeled and cut produce in an airtight bag in the refrigerator and use within 24 hours.

- Wash, core, peel (if not organic), and cut fruit and vegetables into pieces. Flash-freeze by layering the fruit or vegetables in one layer on a baking sheet in the coldest part of the freezer for an hour or until solid. Then store them in an airtight bag in the freezer for up to three months. Use as needed.

Berry Mixer

Prep time: About 3 min • **Blending time:** 1 min • **Yield:** 2 servings

Ingredients	Directions
½ cup cranberry or pomegranate juice	**1** Combine the cranberry or pomegranate juice, lime juice, honey, alcohol, and berries in the blender container.
2 tablespoons fresh lime juice	
2 tablespoons honey	**2** Secure the lid on the container.
2 ounces rum, gin, or vodka	**3** Starting on a low speed and gradually easing toward high, blend the ingredients for 30 seconds. Add ice and pulse for 20 seconds or until ice is evenly mixed in.
¾ cup frozen berries (see Tip)	
¼ cup crushed ice	**4** Pour the smoothie into 2 glasses and enjoy!

Per serving: Calories 193 (From Fat 3); Fat 0g (Saturated 0g); Cholesterol 0mg; Sodium 3mg; Carbohydrate 33g (Dietary Fiber 3g); Protein 1g.

Tip: This drink may be tart tasting, so you can use honey or agave nectar or brown rice syrup to sweeten it to taste.

Vary It! Blueberries, raspberries, strawberries, blackberries, acai berries, and even cherries work well in this mixer.

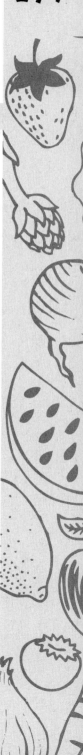

Chapter 17

Blending Vegetable Smoothies

In This Chapter

▶ Drinking your veggies throughout the day

▶ Getting the party started with savory smoothies

*F*ace it: Most people just don't eat enough vegetables. A 2007 study from Johns Hopkins University showed that among US adults, fruit consumption is holding steady, but vegetable consumption is headed down.

So, how many do you need? Some experts say five fruits and vegetables a day. If you're not eating five fruits and vegetables every day, this is an excellent goal to set to start. However, the US Department of Agriculture (USDA) actually recommends two to four servings of fruit and three to five servings of vegetables every day. For optimum health and disease prevention, aim for as many as ten or more servings of fruits and vegetables per day.

What can you do if you're part of that group of people who aren't eating enough veggies? You can start drinking them! Because they include the carbohydrate and fiber along with the nutrients, smoothies give you a feeling of fullness that stays with you longer than juices. The average vegetable smoothie will supply two to three servings of vegetables (or fruit and vegetables), so you get a double or triple hit of these valuable foods with every drink.

Getting a Jump-Start with Breakfast Smoothies

Vegetables at breakfast? Why not? Although the traditional breakfast drink is orange juice, a raw vegetable or green smoothie provides antioxidants and phytonutrients in a convenient and much more digestible form, because the blender has done all the work of breaking down the plant cellulose.

You wake up in the morning dehydrated, with your blood slightly acidic, so raw vegetable smoothies not only feed and nourish your cells, but also rehydrate and help to balance your pH levels.

For morning vegetable smoothies, leafy greens such as spinach, kale, Swiss chard, and fresh herbs are a good choice to blend with carrots, zucchini, or tomatoes and *one* fruit, such as pineapple, mango, kiwi, banana, berries, or cherries.

Yogurt or cottage cheese is a good addition at breakfast, because the protein takes longer to digest. Combining yogurt or cottage cheese with non-starchy vegetables is usually tolerable for people with very sensitive digestive systems, too — so even if you can't tolerate fruit and protein together in the same meal or drink, you may be able to consume vegetables like summer squash, cucumber, tomatoes, broccoli, green beans, and sweet peppers along with yogurt or cottage cheese in a cool vegetable smoothie.

Foods to avoid if you're prone to yeast or viral infections

If you have a yeast infection, if you've recently taken antibiotics, or if you've recently suffered a viral infection (like a cold), avoid the following foods — they feed yeast, bacteria, and viruses:

✔ **All sweet foods:** Sugar, candy, syrups, toppings, ice cream, sweetened desserts, and sweetened breakfast cereals

✔ **All refined grains:** White bread, cakes, cookies, tarts, pies, and baked goods

✔ **Pasta:** Wheat and gluten-free noodles, rice, lasagna, and spaghetti

✔ **Fruits:** All fruits *except* sour fruits, such as pomegranate, acai berries, cranberries, and lemon

✔ **Root vegetables:** Beets, carrots, parsnips, and potatoes

Green Energy Breakfast

Prep time: About 3 min • **Blending time:** 1 min • **Yield:** 2 servings

Ingredients	Directions
1 cucumber	**1** Peel the cucumber and cut into chunks.
2 cups fresh or 1 cup frozen spinach	**2** Chop the spinach into cubes (if using frozen).
½ cup almond milk	
½ cup fresh basil leaves	**3** Combine the milk, cucumber, spinach, basil, yogurt, and hemp seeds or flaxseed in the blender container.
⅔ cup plain low-fat yogurt	
1 tablespoon ground hemp seeds or flaxseed	**4** Secure the lid on the container.
	5 Starting on a low speed and gradually easing toward high, blend the ingredients for 45 seconds or until smooth and no visible pieces of vegetable are in the mixture.
	6 Pour the smoothie into 2 glasses and enjoy!

Per serving: Calories 94 (From Fat 22); Fat 2g (Saturated 0g); Cholesterol 2mg; Sodium 116mg; Carbohydrate 14g (Dietary Fiber 3g); Protein 6g.

Vary It! For a slightly sweeter version, use fresh apple juice or orange juice in place of the almond milk and add 1 peeled and quartered kiwifruit.

Tip: To make thick, Greek-style yogurt, strain plain yogurt through cheesecloth.

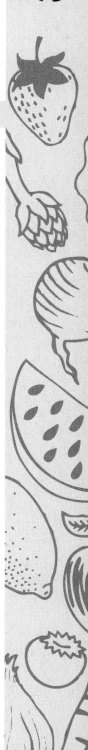

Vita-E

Prep time: About 4 min • **Blending time:** 1 min • **Yield:** 2 servings

Ingredients	Directions
1 red or green bell pepper ½ avocado	*1* Cut the pepper in half. Remove the seeds and membrane, and cut it into chunks.
1¼ cup fresh carrot juice 2 cups fresh chard pieces or spinach	*2* Peel the avocado, remove the stone, and cut into chunks.
3 tablespoons chopped raw almonds 2 tablespoons rolled oats (large-flake oatmeal)	*3* Combine the carrot juice, chard or spinach, pepper, avocado, almonds, oats, and flaxseed in the blender container.
1 tablespoon ground flaxseed	*4* Secure the lid on the container.
	5 Starting on a low speed and gradually easing toward high, blend the ingredients for 45 seconds or until smooth and no visible pieces of vegetable or nuts are in the mixture.
	6 Pour the smoothie into 2 glasses and enjoy!

Per serving: Calories 213 (From Fat 116); Fat 13g (Saturated 2g); Cholesterol 0mg; Sodium 156mg; Carbohydrate 23g (Dietary Fiber 8g); Protein 7g.

Tip: Vitamin E prevents cell damage from free radicals and helps protect against prostate cancer and Alzheimer's disease.

Vary It! If you're juicing the carrots for this smoothie, try adding a parsnip or half a beet to vary the juice.

Tomato Energizer

Prep time: About 4 min • **Blending time:** 1 min • **Yield:** 2 servings

Ingredients	Directions
2 small zucchini	**1** Peel the zucchini and cut into chunks.
1 red or green bell pepper	**2** Cut the pepper in half. Remove the seeds and membrane, and cut it into chunks.
¾ cup fresh tomato juice	
2 tablespoons fresh lemon juice	**3** Combine the tomato juice, lemon juice, parsley, zucchini, tomatoes, pepper, and ginger in the blender container.
¼ cup fresh parsley leaves	
2 medium tomatoes, quartered	**4** Secure the lid on the container.
1 tablespoon fresh grated ginger	**5** Starting on a low speed and gradually easing toward high, blend the ingredients for 45 seconds or until smooth and no visible pieces of vegetable are in the mixture.
	6 Pour the smoothie into 2 glasses and enjoy!

Per serving: Calories 95 (From Fat 8); Fat 1g (Saturated 0g); Cholesterol 0mg; Sodium 23mg; Carbohydrate 21g (Dietary Fiber 5g); Protein 5g.

Vary It! Red pepper adds color and easily substitutes for the green pepper.

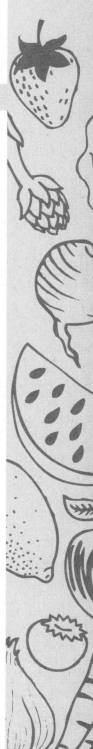

Red Vitality

Prep time: About 4 min • **Blending time:** 1 min • **Yield:** 2 servings

Ingredients	Directions
1 pear	*1* Peel the pear (if not organic) and cut into quarters. Remove the core and seeds.
2 small beets, lightly steamed	
¾ cup fresh carrot juice	*2* Peel the beets and cut into eighths.
2 tablespoons fresh lemon juice	*3* Combine the carrot juice, lemon juice, spinach, tomatoes, pear, and beets in the blender container.
1 cup fresh spinach	
2 medium tomatoes, quartered	*4* Secure the lid on the container.
	5 Starting on a low speed and gradually easing toward high, blend the ingredients for 45 seconds or until smooth and no visible pieces of vegetable are in the mixture.
	6 Pour the smoothie into 2 glasses and enjoy!

Per serving: Calories 141 (From Fat 10); Fat 1g (Saturated 0g); Cholesterol 0mg; Sodium 135mg; Carbohydrate 33g (Dietary Fiber 6g); Protein 1g.

Vary It! You can use an apple, mango, or other whole fruit or a slice of pineapple in place of the pear in this drink.

Serving up Lunch and Dinner Smoothies

The USDA suggests that eating three to five servings of vegetables daily reduces the risk of stroke, type 2 diabetes, cancer, heart disease, and bone loss. Vegetables rich in potassium help to maintain healthy blood pressure, while those high in Vitamin C keep connective tissue, including gums, healthy. Vitamin A in vegetables helps the immune system fight infections and promotes healthy eyes and skin.

An added benefit of vegetables is their low energy density, which means they don't have as many calories, volume for volume, as most other foods. This makes them a great choice for snacks because the fiber in them gives you a satisfied feeling of fullness, helping you resist high-fat or empty-calorie between-meal bites.

For the same reasons, vegetable smoothies also may replace lunch and dinner occasionally. Some weight-loss diet plans suggest that you replace one or two meals a day with a vegetable smoothie, but I recommend that you work with a healthcare professional before starting in on any aggressive weight-loss program.

If you plan to use vegetable smoothies as meal replacements regularly, you'll need to ensure that one meal of the day includes a portion of low-fat protein (chicken, fish or shellfish, nuts, seeds, or legumes) along with raw or cooked vegetables, whole grains, and one serving of fruit.

Cooked legumes (lentils, peas, or beans) make a great lunch or dinner smoothie ingredient because of their plant proteins, which tend to stay with you longer than carbohydrates. The high-fiber content prevents blood sugar levels from rising rapidly and helps lower cholesterol. Legumes are also excellent sources of folate, tryptophan, manganese, and iron.

To use cooked, canned legumes, simply open and spoon into the blender container. You may prefer to drain and rinse canned legumes before adding to the container, but the liquid contains water-soluble nutrients, so I recommend adding it to the liquid ingredients in the smoothie.

All the smoothies in this section are very thick and meant to be eaten with a spoon.

Beans and Carrots

Prep time: About 3 min • **Blending time:** 1 min • **Yield:** 2 servings

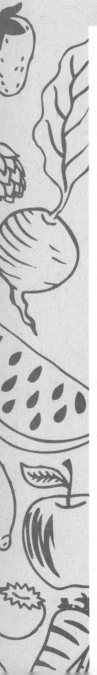

Ingredients	Directions
1 cucumber	*1* Peel the cucumber and cut it into chunks.
1 apple	*2* Peel the apple (if not organic) and cut into quarters. Remove the core and seeds.
1 cup fresh carrot juice	
1 cup cooked lentils or lima beans	*3* Combine the carrot juice, cucumber, lentils or lima beans, and apple in the blender container.
	4 Secure the lid on the container.
	5 Starting on a low speed and gradually easing toward high, blend the ingredients for 45 seconds or until smooth and no visible pieces of vegetable are in the mixture.
	6 Pour the smoothie into 2 glasses and enjoy!

Per serving: Calories 188 (From Fat 8); Fat 1g (Saturated 0g); Cholesterol 0mg; Sodium 65mg; Carbohydrate 38g (Dietary Fiber 10g); Protein 10g.

Vary It! Green, red, or brown lentils may be used in this recipe. You can use any cooked, canned bean such as navy beans, lima beans, or chickpeas.

Greek Salad

Prep time: About 3 min • **Blending time:** 1 min • **Yield:** 2 servings

Ingredients	Directions
3 medium tomatoes	**1** Remove stem if still attached and coarsely chop the tomatoes.
1 cucumber	
1 avocado	**2** Peel the cucumber and cut it into chunks.
½ cup fresh apple juice	
1 or 2 tablespoons chopped sweet onion, or to taste	**3** Peel and seed the avocado and cut the flesh into chunks.
¼ cup feta cheese cubes, optional	**4** Combine the apple juice, tomatoes, cucumber, avocado, onion, feta, and dill in the blender container.
¼ teaspoon fresh chopped dill	
	5 Secure the lid on the container.
	6 Starting on a low speed and gradually easing toward high, blend the ingredients for 45 seconds or until smooth and no visible pieces of vegetable are in the mixture.
	7 Pour the smoothie into 2 glasses and enjoy!

Per serving: Calories 232 (From Fat 108); Fat 12g (Saturated 1g); Cholesterol 0mg; Sodium 9mg; Carbohydrate 31g (Dietary Fiber 6g); Protein 6g.

Tip: Adding feta cheese makes this a really thick drink with authentic Greek flavor. If you're unsure about this ingredient — or any ingredient that you're trying for the first time — add a small amount, blend, and taste before adding more.

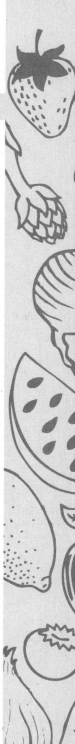

Spiced Parsnip

Prep time: About 3 min • **Blending time:** 1 min • **Yield:** 2 servings

Ingredients	Directions
3 lightly steamed or cooked parsnips	**1** Cut the parsnips into chunks.
1 cup fresh apple juice 1 cup cooked chickpeas ¼ cup chopped walnuts ¼ teaspoon ground cinnamon ⅛ teaspoon cayenne pepper (or to taste)	**2** Combine the apple juice, parsnips, chickpeas, walnuts, cinnamon, and cayenne pepper in the blender container.
	3 Secure the lid on the container.
	4 Starting on a low speed and gradually easing toward high, blend the ingredients for 45 seconds or until smooth and no visible pieces of vegetable are in the mixture.
	5 Pour the smoothie into 2 glasses and enjoy!

Per serving: Calories 486 (From Fat 115); Fat 13g (Saturated 1g); Cholesterol 0mg; Sodium 34mg; Carbohydrate 86g (Dietary Fiber 17g); Protein 13g.

Tip: Make extra vegetables at dinner — steamed, roasted, or simmered. Freeze them or store them in the refrigerator and use in smoothies the next day.

Berry Broccoli

Prep time: About 3 min • **Blending time:** 1 min • **Yield:** 2 servings

Ingredients	Directions
½ cup fresh carrot juice	**1** Combine the carrot juice, applesauce, yogurt, broccoli or broccoli rabe, blueberries, and nutmeg in the blender container.
½ cup applesauce	
½ cup plain low-fat yogurt	
1 cup lightly steamed broccoli or broccoli rabe	**2** Secure the lid on the container.
1 cup frozen blueberries	**3** Starting on a low speed and gradually easing toward high, blend the ingredients for 45 seconds or until smooth and no visible pieces of vegetable are in the mixture.
¼ teaspoon nutmeg	
	4 Pour the smoothie into 2 glasses and enjoy!

Per serving: Calories 162 (From Fat 18); Fat 2g (Saturated 1g); Cholesterol 4mg; Sodium 96mg; Carbohydrate 33g (Dietary Fiber 4g); Protein 6g.

Tip: You can use raw broccoli in smoothies, but the texture and taste is better if it's lightly steamed or simmered first.

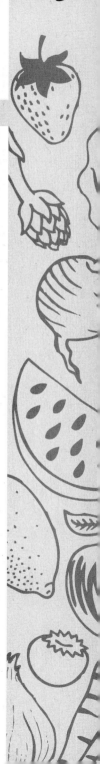

Coconut Green

Prep time: About 3 min • **Blending time:** 1 min • **Yield:** 2 servings

Ingredients	Directions
1 cucumber	*1* Peel the cucumber and cut it into chunks.
1 cup coconut or almond milk	*2* Combine the coconut or almond milk, cucumber, spinach, lentils or lima beans, and coconut oil in the blender container.
2 cups fresh spinach	
1 cup cooked lentils or lima beans	*3* Secure the lid on the container.
1 heaping tablespoon coconut oil	*4* Starting on a low speed and gradually easing toward high, blend the ingredients for 45 seconds or until smooth and no visible pieces of vegetable are in the mixture.
	5 Pour the smoothie into 2 glasses and enjoy!

Per serving: Calories 415 (From Fat 284); Fat 32g (Saturated 27g); Cholesterol 0mg; Sodium 42mg; Carbohydrate 27g (Dietary Fiber 11g); Protein 13g.

Tip: Using coconut oil in smoothies adds good fats and lauric acid, which helps fight harmful bacteria. The fats stay with you longer than carbohydrates, giving you the feeling of being full.

Immunizing Soup

Prep time: About 3 min • **Blending time:** 1 min • **Yield:** 2 servings

Ingredients	Directions
1 cup fresh carrot juice 1 cup fresh or frozen spinach, chopped 1 cup cooked kidney or pinto beans ¼ sweet onion 1 tablespoon coconut oil ¼ teaspoon chopped fresh rosemary	*1* Combine the carrot juice, spinach, beans, onion, coconut oil, and rosemary in the blender container. *2* Secure the lid on the container. *3* Starting on a low speed and gradually easing toward high, blend the ingredients for 45 seconds or until smooth and no visible pieces of vegetable are in the mixture. *4* To heat the soup, warm in a saucepan over medium-high heat or if using a high-performance blender, blend on high for 1 or 2 minutes or until the soup is hot. *5* Pour the smoothie into 2 bowls or glasses and enjoy!

Per serving: *Calories 244 (From Fat 63); Fat 7g (Saturated 6g); Cholesterol 0mg; Sodium 227mg; Carbohydrate 34g (Dietary Fiber 8g); Protein 11g.*

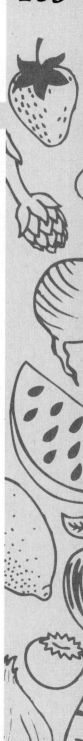

Lentil Soup

Prep time: About 3 min • **Blending time:** 1 min • **Yield:** 2 servings

Ingredients	Directions
1 orange	*1* Peel the orange and break into sections. Remove the seeds.
1 mango	
1 cup fresh orange juice	*2* Peel the mango, remove the stone, and cut into chunks.
2 tablespoons fresh lime juice	*3* Combine the orange juice, lime juice, spinach, lentils or lima beans, orange, mango, and whey powder in the blender container.
2 cups fresh spinach	
1 cup cooked lentils or lima beans	*4* Secure the lid on the container.
2 tablespoons whey powder	*5* Starting on a low speed and gradually easing toward high, blend the ingredients for 45 seconds or until smooth and no visible pieces of vegetable are in the mixture.
	6 Pour into a saucepan and heat over medium-high heat for 3 to 4 minutes or until heated; or pour into a microwave-safe bowl and microwave on high for 1 minute or until hot.
	7 Pour the smoothie into 2 bowls or glasses and enjoy!

Per serving: Calories 317 (From Fat 13); Fat 1g (Saturated 0g); Cholesterol 0mg; Sodium 91mg; Carbohydrate 64g (Dietary Fiber 13g); Protein 17g.

Tip: If you own a high-performance blender, skip Step 6 and run the machine on high for 4 to 6 minutes or until the soup is hot.

Vary It! Any dark leafy green (chard, beet tops, collard greens, or kale) may be substituted for the spinach. You can use chopped frozen greens in this smoothie if you don't have fresh on hand.

Vegetable Soup

Prep time: About 3 min • **Blending time:** 1 min • **Heating time:** 1–5 min • **Yield:** 2 servings

Ingredients	Directions
½ **cucumber**	**1** Peel the cucumber and cut it and the carrot into chunks.
1 carrot	
1 cup vegetable or chicken broth	**2** Combine the broth, tomatoes, chard or kale, cilantro or parsley, cucumber, and carrot in the blender container.
3 medium tomatoes, cored and quartered	
½ **cup cilantro or parsley**	**3** Secure the lid on the container.
	4 Starting on a low speed and gradually easing toward high, blend the ingredients for 45 seconds or until smooth and no visible pieces of vegetable are in the mixture.
	5 Pour into a saucepan and heat over medium-high heat for 5 to 10 minutes or until carrot is soft; or pour into a microwave-safe bowl and microwave on high for 1 minute or until hot.
	6 Pour the soup into 2 bowls and enjoy!

Per serving: Calories 98 (From Fat 14); Fat 2g (Saturated 0g); Cholesterol 0mg; Sodium 557mg; Carbohydrate 21g (Dietary Fiber 5g); Protein 5g.

Vary It! If you want a chunkier soup, pulse for 10 to 20 seconds in Step 4.

Tip: If you own a high-performance blender, skip Step 5 and run the machine on high for 4 to 6 minutes or until the soup is hot.

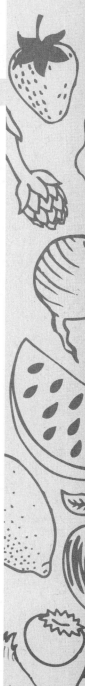

Bean Soup

Prep time: About 3 min • **Blending time:** 1 min • **Heating time:** 1–5 min • **Yield:** 2 servings

Ingredients	Directions
2 green onions	*1* Cut the onions, celery, and carrot into chunks.
2 celery stalks	
1 carrot	*2* Combine the broth, onions, celery, beans, carrot, and savory or thyme in the blender container.
1 cup vegetable or chicken broth	
1 cup cooked kidney or navy beans	*3* Secure the lid on the container.
1 tablespoon fresh savory or thyme leaves	*4* Starting on a low speed and gradually easing toward high, blend the ingredients for 45 seconds or until smooth and no visible pieces of vegetable are in the mixture.
	5 Pour into a saucepan and heat over medium-high heat for 5 to 10 minutes or until vegetables are soft; or pour into a microwave-safe bowl and microwave on high for 1 minute or until hot.
	6 Pour the soup into 2 bowls, and enjoy!

Per serving: Calories 155 (From Fat 9); Fat 1g (Saturated 0g); Cholesterol 0mg; Sodium 574mg; Carbohydrate 29g (Dietary Fiber 8g); Protein 10g.

Vary It! If you want a chunkier soup, pulse for 10 to 20 seconds in Step 4.

Tip: If you own a high-performance blender, skip Step 5 and run the machine on high for 4 to 6 minutes or until the soup is hot.

Cabbage Slaw

Prep time: About 3 min • **Blending time:** 1 min • **Yield:** 2 servings

Ingredients	Directions
2 green onions	*1* Cut the onions, celery, and carrot into chunks.
2 celery stalks	
1 carrot	*2* Peel the apple (if not organic) and cut into quarters. Remove the core and seeds.
1 apple	
1 cup fresh carrot juice	*3* Combine the carrot juice, yogurt, onions, cabbage, celery, carrot, apple, walnuts, and thyme in the blender container.
½ cup plain yogurt	
1 cup chopped red or green cabbage	
2 tablespoons chopped walnuts	*4* Secure the lid on the container.
1 tablespoon fresh thyme leaves	*5* Starting on a low speed and gradually easing toward high, blend the ingredients for 45 seconds or until smooth and no visible pieces of vegetable are in the mixture.
	6 Pour the smoothie into 2 glasses and enjoy!

Per serving: Calories 190 (From Fat 57); Fat 6g (Saturated 1g); Cholesterol 4mg; Sodium 183mg; Carbohydrate 30g (Dietary Fiber 5g); Protein 7g.

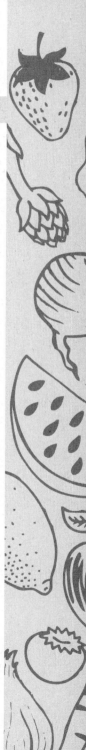

Snacking on Superfood Smoothies

If you find yourself reaching for a liquid fruit or vegetable drink instead of empty calories in the form of pastry or fast, packaged snacks or soda, you're on your way toward a healthier body. Now it's time to fine-tune those smoothie snacks by blending up ingredients that power your activities and at the same time, pack a wallop for your heart, your brain, and your immune system.

Vibrant raw vegetables, lightly sweetened with frozen strawberries, banana chunks, or peach slices and tweaked with super nutrients are perfect for sipping on the go. Smoothie snacking between meals can actually keep you from overindulging in calorie-rich, sweet, or salty bites, and the soluble fiber of fruit and vegetables stays in your tummy longer, making you feel full and steadily releasing glucose, giving you long-term energy. Soluble fiber also benefits your heart by helping to lower LDL (bad) cholesterol.

Black Immunity

Prep time: About 1 min • **Blending time:** 1 min • **Yield:** 2 servings

Ingredients	Directions
1 cup nonsweetened cranberry juice	**1** Combine the cranberry juice, berries, cabbage, beans, carrot and chocolate in the blender container.
1 cup fresh or frozen blackberries, blueberries, raspberries, or a mixture	
	2 Secure the lid on the container.
1 cup shredded red cabbage (see tip)	**3** Starting on a low speed and gradually easing toward high, blend the ingredients for 45 seconds or until smooth and no visible pieces of vegetable are in the mixture.
½ cup cooked black beans	
1 small carrot, chopped	
1 tablespoon powdered dark chocolate cocoa	**4** Pour the smoothie into 2 glasses and enjoy!

Per serving: Calories 170 (From Fat 7); Fat 1g (Saturated 0g); Cholesterol 0mg; Sodium 60mg; Carbohydrate 39g (Dietary Fiber 9g); Protein 6g.

Tip: Here is where a high-performance blender outshines all traditional blenders, but if you don't own one powerful enough to liquefy raw vegetables, cook the cabbage and carrot before blending. In a saucepan, cover cabbage and carrot with water and simmer over medium-high heat for 2 or 3 minutes or until crisp-tender. Cool before adding to the other ingredients in the blender. As promised, this smoothie is black and brimming with immune-boosting anthocyanins.

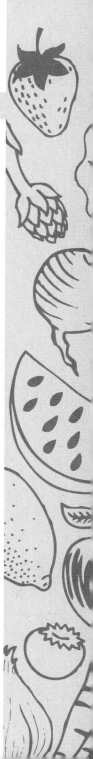

Orange Ade

Prep time: About 1 min • **Blending time:** 1 min • **Yield:** 2 servings

Ingredients	Directions
2 mangoes	*1* Peel and stone the mangoes and chop the flesh.
1 cup fresh carrot juice	*2* Combine the carrot juice, mangoes, broccoli, almond butter, and coconut oil in the blender container.
1 cup chopped broccoli	
1 tablespoon almond butter	
1 tablespoon coconut oil	*3* Secure the lid on the container.
	4 Starting on a low speed and gradually easing toward high, blend the ingredients for 45 seconds or until smooth and no visible pieces of vegetable are in the mixture.
	5 Pour the smoothie into 2 glasses and enjoy!

Per serving: Calories 359 (From Fat 116); Fat 13g (Saturated 7g); Cholesterol 0mg; Sodium 121mg; Carbohydrate 62g (Dietary Fiber 7g); Protein 7g.

Tip: Raw is always the optimal smoothie ingredient, but if the taste of broccoli or cabbage is too strong, start by lightly simmering or steaming it before adding to the blender. With time, your taste buds will become adjusted to the vibrant flavor of raw vegetables.

Blue-Green Brain

Prep time: About 2 min • **Blending time:** 1 min • **Yield:** 2 servings

Ingredients	Directions
1 avocado	*1* Peel and stone the avocado and chop the flesh.
1 cup coconut water	
1 cup chopped red cabbage	*2* Combine the coconut water, avocado, cabbage, blueberries, and green tea in the blender container.
1 cup fresh or frozen blueberries	
1 tablespoon macha or powdered green tea	*3* Secure the lid on the container.
	4 Starting on a low speed and gradually easing toward high, blend the ingredients for 45 seconds or until smooth and no visible pieces of vegetable are in the mixture.
	5 Pour the smoothie into 2 glasses and enjoy!

Per serving: Calories 197 (From Fat 104); Fat 12g (Saturated 1g); Cholesterol 0mg; Sodium 14mg; Carbohydrate 25g (Dietary Fiber 5g); Protein 4g.

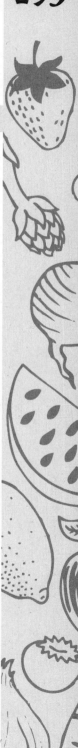

Blue Almond Joy

Prep time: About 2 min • **Blending time:** 1 min • **Yield:** 2 servings

Ingredients	Directions
1 medium beet	*1* Trim beet and grate.
1 cup fresh carrot juice	
1 cup fresh or frozen acai or blueberries	*2* Combine the carrot juice, beet, acai or blueberries, and almonds in the blender container. Open the capsules and squeeze the vitamin E into the blender container.
¼ cup unsalted raw almonds	
2 capsules Vitamin E	*3* Secure the lid on the container.
	4 Starting on a low speed and gradually easing toward high, blend the ingredients for 45 seconds or until smooth and no visible pieces of vegetable are in the mixture.
	5 Pour the smoothie into 2 glasses and enjoy!

Per serving: Calories 183 (From Fat 75); Fat 8g (Saturated 1g); Cholesterol 0mg; Sodium 110mg; Carbohydrate 24g (Dietary Fiber 4g); Protein 6g.

Calming Cocktail

Prep time: About 2 min • **Blending time:** 1 min • **Yield:** 2 servings

Ingredients	Directions
1 cup almond milk	*1* Combine the almond milk, kale, berries, basil, dates, banana, and bee pollen in the blender container.
1 cup chopped kale or spinach	
1 cup fresh or frozen berries	*2* Secure the lid on the container.
¼ cup fresh basil leaves	*3* Starting on a low speed and gradually easing toward high, blend the ingredients for 45 seconds or until smooth and no visible pieces of vegetable are in the mixture.
¼ cup chopped and pitted dates	
1 fresh or frozen banana	
1 tablespoon bee pollen	*4* Pour the smoothie into 2 glasses and enjoy!

Per serving: Calories 210 (From Fat 20); Fat 2g (Saturated 0g); Cholesterol 0mg; Sodium 76mg; Carbohydrate 48g (Dietary Fiber 6g); Protein 4g.

Tip: If you're using a traditional blender, try combining the almond milk and the dates in the blender container and set aside for 10 minutes to soften the dates. Add remaining ingredients and continue with Step 2.

Vary It! All deep green, leafy vegetables like spinach, Swiss chard, and, of course, kale may be used in these recipes. Of course, baby leaves are tender and milder in taste than their mature counterparts.

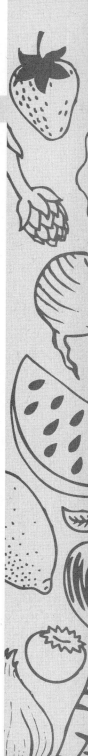

De-Stresser

Prep time: About 2 min • **Blending time:** 1 min • **Yield:** 2 servings

Ingredients	Directions
1 cup almond milk	**1** Combine the almond milk, broccoli, berries, yogurt, and Brewers' yeast in the blender container.
1 cup chopped cooked broccoli	
1 cup fresh or frozen berries	**2** Secure the lid on the container.
½ cup plain yogurt	**3** Starting on a low speed and gradually easing toward high, blend the ingredients for 45 seconds or until smooth and no visible pieces of vegetable are in the mixture.
1 tablespoon Brewers' Yeast	
	4 Pour the smoothie into 2 glasses and enjoy!

Per serving: Calories 151 (From Fat 23); Fat 3g (Saturated 1g); Cholesterol 4mg; Sodium 158mg; Carbohydrate 27g (Dietary Fiber 5g); Protein 9g.

Socializing with Vegetable Mocktail and Cocktail Smoothies

Using vegetable smoothies at social gatherings is just plain smart. You want a slightly sweet and pleasing drink to share with friends, so these nonalcoholic and spiked cocktails are not only delicious but good for you. Table 17-1 lists vegetables that work well for party smoothies, tells you how much to use, and outlines what they'll do for your body.

Table 17-1	Vegetables for Party Smoothies	
Vegetable	*How Much to Add*	*Benefits*
Leafy greens	1 to 2 cups, torn	Provides vitamins A and K, folate, calcium, and folate; turns the drink green or brown
Broccoli	1 to 2 cups, coarsely chopped and steamed or simmered	Provides fiber, potassium, calcium, folate, magnesium, and vitamins C and A; has anticancer properties
Tomatoes	1 to 4, quartered	Adds vitamin C, lycopene, and lutein (for eye health); thins a thick smoothie
Carrots	1 to 3, cut in chunks	Provide vitamins A and C and lutein (for eyes); has anti-cancer properties
Avocados	1 to 2, peeled, stoned, cut in chunks	A good source of folate, vitamin E, potassium, and omega fatty acids; adds thickness and fats
Beets	1 to 3, peeled, cut in chunks	Provides iron, potassium, and magnesium; is a blood and liver tonic; turns the drink (and your urine) pink or red
Asparagus	2 to 6 stalks, cut in chunks	Provides potassium, folate, vitamin K, and other phytonutrients
Cabbage	1 to 2 cups, coarsely chopped	Provides calcium, magnesium, potassium, and vitamins C, K, and A; fights breast and prostate cancer

Minted Carrot Mocktail

Prep time: About 4 min • **Blending time:** 1 min • **Yield:** 2 servings

Ingredients	Directions
2 mangoes	**1** Peel the mangoes and remove the stones. Cut the mangoes and pineapple slices into chunks.
2 slices pineapple, ½-inch thick	
1 carrot, lightly steamed	**2** Cut the carrot into chunks.
¾ cup fresh carrot juice	**3** Combine the carrot juice, lemon juice, mangoes, pineapple, carrot, and chopped mint in the blender container.
2 tablespoons fresh lemon juice	
2 tablespoons chopped fresh mint	**4** Secure the lid on the container.
2 to 4 fresh mint leaves for garnish (optional)	**5** Starting on a low speed and gradually easing toward high, blend the ingredients for 45 seconds or until smooth and no visible pieces of vegetable are in the mixture.
	6 Pour the smoothie into 2 glasses, garnish with fresh mint leaves (if using), and enjoy!

Per serving: Calories 204 (From Fat 9); Fat 1g (Saturated 0g); Cholesterol 0mg; Sodium 73mg; Carbohydrate 52g (Dietary Fiber 6g); Protein 3g.

Spicy Tomato Mocktail

Prep time: About 4 min • **Blending time:** 1 min • **Yield:** 2 servings

Ingredients	Directions
1 apple	**1** Peel the apple (if not organic) and cut into quarters. Remove the core and seeds.
¾ cup fresh carrot juice	
2 tablespoons fresh lime juice	**2** Cut the celery stalks and pineapple slices into chunks.
4 medium tomatoes, quartered	**3** Combine the carrot juice, lime juice, tomatoes, celery, pineapple, apple, hot pepper, and cilantro.
2 stalks celery	
2 slices pineapple, ½ inch thick	**4** Secure the lid on the container.
½ to 1 jalapeno pepper	**5** Starting on a low speed and gradually easing toward high, blend the ingredients for 45 seconds or until smooth and no visible pieces of vegetable are in the mixture.
2 tablespoons chopped fresh cilantro	
2 to 4 fresh cilantro leaves for garnish (optional)	
	6 Pour the smoothie into 2 glasses, garnish with fresh cilantro leaves (if using), and enjoy!

Per serving: Calories 161 (From Fat 14); Fat 2g (Saturated 0g); Cholesterol 0mg; Sodium 124mg; Carbohydrate 39g (Dietary Fiber 6g); Protein 4g.

Tip: Rim the edges of the glasses with coarse salt. Combine ½ cup coarse salt and 1 tablespoon fresh, chopped parsley, thyme, or cilantro. Tip into a shallow dish or saucer. Run a wedge of lime or lemon around the edges of the glasses. Turn glasses upside down and set into the herbed salt. Twist to secure salt to the rim of the glasses and remove. Turn the right side up and fill with the smoothie mixture.

Carrot Mock Mimosa

Prep time: About 3 min • **Blending time:** 1 min • **Yield:** 2 servings

Ingredients	Directions
2 slices pineapple, ½-inch thick	**1** Cut the pineapple slices into chunks.
½ cup fresh carrot juice ½ cup fresh orange juice	**2** Combine the carrot juice, orange juice, pineapple, and carrots in the blender container.
2 carrots, lightly steamed Ice	**3** Secure the lid on the container.
½ cup club soda	**4** Starting on a low speed and gradually easing toward high, blend the ingredients for 45 seconds or until smooth and no visible pieces of vegetable are in the mixture.
	5 Fill 2 tall glasses with ice halfway. Pour the smoothie into the glasses, about three-quarters full. Add club soda and enjoy!

Per serving: Calories 103 (From Fat 4); Fat 0g (Saturated 0g); Cholesterol 0mg; Sodium 72mg; Carbohydrate 24g (Dietary Fiber 3g); Protein 2g.

Tip: You can use raw carrots if you want, but cooked carrots make a smoother drink.

Tip: Garnish with orange slices if you wish. The ice may be omitted if you want.

No-jito

Prep time: About 4 min • **Blending time:** 1 min • **Yield:** 2 servings

Ingredients	Directions
1 avocado	*1* Cut the avocado in half, remove the stone, and peel. Cut the avocado and celery into chunks.
1 stalk celery	
1 apple	*2* Peel the apple (if not organic) and cut into quarters. Remove the core and seeds.
2 cups fresh or 1 cup frozen spinach	
¾ cup fresh carrot juice	*3* Chop the spinach if using frozen.
¼ cup fresh lime juice	*4* Combine the carrot juice, lime juice, spinach, celery, avocado, apple, and chopped mint in the blender container.
2 tablespoons chopped fresh mint	
2 to 4 fresh mint leaves for garnish (optional)	*5* Secure the lid on the container.
	6 Starting on a low speed and gradually easing toward high, blend the ingredients for 45 seconds or until smooth and no visible pieces of vegetable are in the mixture.
	7 Pour the smoothie into 2 glasses, garnish with fresh mint leaves (if using), and enjoy!

Per serving: Calories 215 (From Fat 117); Fat 13g (Saturated 3g); Cholesterol 0mg; Sodium 97mg; Carbohydrate 27g (Dietary Fiber 11g); Protein 5g.

Vary It! This makes a thick smoothie. You can thin it by using 1 cup carrot juice or by using ½ avocado.

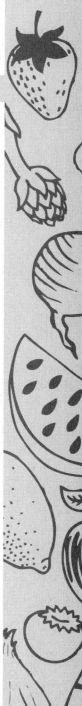

Red Velvet

Prep time: About 4 min • **Blending time:** 1 min • **Yield:** 4 servings

Ingredients	Directions
½ **avocado**	**1** Cut the avocado and red pepper into chunks.
½ **red pepper**	
1 **apple**	**2** Peel the apple (if not organic) and cut into quarters. Remove the core and seeds.
2 **small beets, lightly steamed**	
1 **cup almond milk**	**3** Peel the beets and cut into chunks.
2 **ounces vodka, light rum, or gin**	**4** Combine the almond milk, alcohol, avocado, pepper, apple, beets, nuts, cocoa powder, and honey in the blender container.
¼ **cup cashews or macadamia nuts**	
2 **tablespoons cocoa powder**	**5** Secure the lid on the container.
1 **to 2 tablespoons honey (or to taste)**	**6** Starting on a low speed and gradually easing toward high, blend the ingredients for 45 seconds or until smooth and no visible pieces of vegetable are in the mixture.
1 **cup frozen strawberries**	
	7 Add frozen strawberries and pulse for 30 seconds or until blended into the mixture.
	8 Pour the smoothie into 4 glasses, and enjoy!

Per serving: Calories 206 (From Fat 77); Fat 9g (Saturated 2g); Cholesterol 0mg; Sodium 73mg; Carbohydrate 25g (Dietary Fiber 6g); Protein 4g.

Vary It! The avocado makes this a thick drink. You can omit it for a thinner smoothie.

Grape Cocktail

Prep time: About 4 min • **Blending time:** 1 min • **Yield:** 2 servings

Ingredients	Directions
½ **avocado**	*1* Peel and cut the flesh of the avocado into chunks. Tightly wrap and refrigerate the remaining half.
1 cup grape juice	
1 cup blueberries	*2* Combine the grape juice, avocado, blueberries, and cabbage in the blender container.
2 cups chopped red cabbage	
1 cup frozen red grapes	*3* Secure the lid on the container.
2 ounces vodka, light rum, or gin	
	4 Starting on a low speed and gradually easing toward high, blend the ingredients for 45 seconds or until smooth and no visible pieces of vegetable are in the mixture.
	5 Add frozen grapes and pulse for 30 seconds or until blended into the mixture.
	6 Pour the smoothie into 2 glasses, add 1 ounce of alcohol to each glass, stir, and enjoy!

Per serving: Calories 320 (From Fat 65); Fat 7g (Saturated 1g); Cholesterol 0mg; Sodium 52mg; Carbohydrate 99g (Dietary Fiber 16g); Protein 7g.

Vary It! Ice thickens and chills smoothies. Add ½ cup crushed ice in Step 5 if desired.

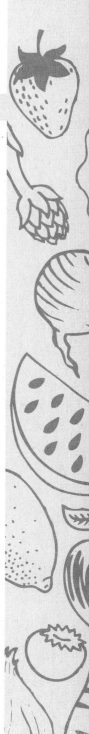

Crème de Cocao

Prep time: About 4 min • **Blending time:** 1 min • **Yield:** 2 servings

Ingredients	Directions
½ avocado	*1* Peel and cut the flesh of the avocado into chunks.
1 cup coconut cream or coconut milk	*2* Combine the coconut cream or milk, avocado, and cabbage in the blender container.
2 cups chopped green cabbage, lightly steamed	*3* Secure the lid on the container.
1 cup frozen green grapes	*4* Starting on a low speed and gradually easing toward high, blend the ingredients for 45 seconds or until smooth and no visible pieces of vegetable are in the mixture.
2 ounces vodka, light rum, or gin	*5* Add the frozen grapes and pulse for 30 seconds or until blended into the mixture.
	6 Pour the smoothie into 2 glasses, clean the container and lid.
	7 Add 1 ounce of alcohol to each glass, stir, and enjoy!

Per serving: Calories 493 (From Fat 298); Fat 33g (Saturated 25g); Cholesterol 0mg; Sodium 89mg; Carbohydrate 34g (Dietary Fiber 9g); Protein 7g.

Vary It! Ice thickens and chills smoothies. Add ½ cup crushed ice in Step 5 if desired.

Cucumber Gin

Prep time: About 4 min • **Blending time:** 1 min • **Yield:** 2 servings

Ingredients	Directions
1 cup tonic water 2 cups chopped cucumber 2 ounces vodka, light rum, or gin 1 cup frozen green grapes	*1* Combine the tonic water, cucumber, and alcohol in the blender container.
	2 Secure the lid on the container.
	3 Starting on a low speed and gradually easing toward high, blend the ingredients for 45 seconds or until smooth and no visible pieces of vegetable are in the mixture.
	4 Add the frozen grapes and pulse for 30 seconds or until blended into the mixture.
	5 Pour the smoothie into 2 glasses and enjoy!

Per serving: Calories 180 (From Fat 6); Fat 1g (Saturated 0g); Cholesterol 0mg; Sodium 9mg; Carbohydrate 28g (Dietary Fiber 2g); Protein 1g.

Vary It! Ice thickens and chills smoothies. Add ¼ cup crushed ice in Step 4 if desired.

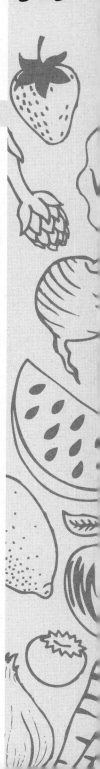

Adding smart foods to smoothies

Ingredients that feed the brain and help reduce stress are those that are rich in omega-3 fatty acids, antioxidants, and vitamins C, B complex, and E. Suffering from anxiety, depression, or tension may be part of living in today's modern society, but a healthy diet and exercise plan can help you avoid many of the stressful side effects of life. Here is a list of the very best brain and immunity foods and stress-busters to add to smoothies.

✔ **Blue, black, and acai berries:** They reduce the aging and brain-cell damaging effects of oxidative stress. Add ½ cup fresh, frozen, or freeze-dried.

✔ **Coconut oil and avocados:** Their medium chain and monounsaturated fats contribute to healthy blood flow, and they also help lower blood pressure, making them beneficial to a healthy brain. Add a quarter fresh avocado and up to 1 tablespoon coconut oil.

✔ **Dark chocolate:** High in antioxidants and caffeine, it helps you concentrate and stimulates the production of endorphins. Add ½ ounce melted dark (79 percent or higher cacao) chocolate or 1 tablespoon powdered, unsweetened dark chocolate.

✔ **Gingko biloba:** It protects and helps repair damaged nerve cells so that memory is improved and feelings of depression are lifted. Add ½ teaspoon powdered or the contents of one capsule.

✔ **Green tea:** Its antioxidant properties help shield brain cells from ravage caused by oxidation. Brew 1 cup fresh green tea, cool, and use as the liquid in smoothies or add 1 tablespoon powdered green tea or macha.

✔ **Legumes:** Because of their soluble fiber, they stabilize glucose (blood sugar) levels, providing a steady source of energy to the brain. Lentils and legumes are high in folate. Add ½ cup cooked lentils or legumes.

✔ **Nuts and seeds:** Their high vitamin E and B2 makes them beneficial in preventing cognitive decline and bolstering the immune system during times of stress. Add ¼ cup nuts and 1 tablespoon of seeds or nut butter.

✔ **Oatmeal:** Its soluble fiber lowers cholesterol levels, and its antioxidants and B1 help keep cells healthy. Add 2 to 4 tablespoons large flake, old-fashioned oatmeal.

✔ **Rhodiola rosea:** It has been proven to have the ability to relieve depression and improve memory and focus. Add ½ teaspoon powdered or empty one capsule.

✔ **Rosemary:** A powerful antioxidant, and its carnosic acid can protect the brain from stroke and neuro-degeneration by toxins and free radicals. Add ¼ to ½ teaspoon chopped fresh.

✔ **Spinach:** High in folate and vitamin C, spinach helps support your nervous system, lowers blood pressure, and may help lift depression. Both vitamin C and magnesium help lower the stress hormone cortisol. Add 1 cup chopped fresh or frozen.

Chapter 18

Creating Dairy Smoothies

This chapter is all about using milk and dairy products in smoothies. If you're lactose intolerant, you may want to substitute lactose-free milk or skip to the next chapter, because every one of the drinks in this chapter is made with milk or products derived from milk.

Because they're made from milk, dairy products — cheese, yogurt, ice cream, cream, crème fraîche, sour cream, and buttermilk — are good sources of calcium and protein. Dairy products aren't limited to cow's milk; they include products from all the various animal milk sources, including sheep and goat.

Why add dairy products to your smoothies? Because they're a great way to increase your calcium and protein intake while you're getting your fruits and vegetables.

Go to www.dummies.com/extras/juicingsmoothies for some dessert recipes.

Starting Your Day with Breakfast and Snack Smoothies

For vitamin- and mineral-enriched breakfast and snack smoothies, choose your milk or milk product and get blending. Because of the protein in milk and milk products, dairy smoothies have staying power, which makes them perfect in the morning for breakfast or midmorning snacks.

Try making these recipes in the morning for breakfast and then bring the remaining serving to work as a midmorning snack. Be sure to fill the glass jar or container as close to the top as possible to reduce exposure to air. Cover tightly and keep in the refrigerator until you're ready to enjoy it on your midmorning break, while all your co-workers are loading up on bagels, donuts, and vending-machine food.

You can use any of the types of liquid milk in these smoothies: whole, 2 percent, 1 percent, or skim milk; buttermilk; or sheep or goat milk. See the nearby sidebar for more on choosing milk for dairy smoothies.

How to choose milk for dairy smoothies

Milk is milk, right? Sort of. There are several different forms of milk, and they all can be used as the liquid ingredient in smoothies, but each has different properties and, of course, nutrients, not to mention fat, and each produces a slightly different texture and thickness in the drink. Here are the most popular forms of milk and what you can expect from them in smoothies:

✔ **Liquid cow's milk:** At supermarkets, you buy milk that has been *pasteurized* (heated for safety) and *homogenized* (the butterfat broken down into small particles so it doesn't float to the top), and it comes in 4 basic forms. Whole milk has 3.25 percent butterfat, which gives body to smoothies and slows down digestion so that you feel full longer. Reduced-fat milk is available in 2 percent, 1 percent, and nonfat (skim). As the butterfat is removed, the milk gets thinner, which makes smoothies made with reduced-fat milk thinner than those made with whole milk.

✔ **Buttermilk:** Although it's a by-product of making butter, buttermilk does not actually contain butter. It has a rich and creamy texture, so smoothies made with buttermilk are thick, but it contains less fat than whole milk (about 1 percent).

✔ **Powdered milk:** Any liquid milk, including buttermilk, can be evaporated to a dry powder and sold as powdered milk. You can add 1 to 3 tablespoons of powdered milk for a thicker smoothie, or whisk 3 tablespoons with 1 cup of water and use it as the liquid.

✔ **Evaporated milk:** Evaporated milk is made by evaporating about half the water in whole or reduced-fat milk and processing it. Smoothies made with evaporated milk are thicker and slightly sweeter than those made with liquid milk.

✔ **Sweetened condensed milk:** In sweetened condensed milk, whole milk and sugar are heated until about 60 percent of the water evaporates, creating a syrupy thick mixture. Because ½ cup contains a whopping 532 calories, it's only added to dessert smoothies by the tablespoon per serving.

Cashew Butter and Strawberries

Prep time: About 3 min • **Blending time:** 1 min • **Yield:** 2 servings

Ingredients	Directions
1 cup 1 percent or 2 percent milk	**1** Combine the milk, yogurt, banana, strawberries, cashew or peanut butter, and sesame seeds in the blender container.
1 cup fruit-on-the-bottom yogurt	
4 chunks frozen banana or 1 fresh banana	**2** Secure the lid on the container.
1 cup fresh or frozen strawberries	**3** Starting on a low speed and gradually easing toward high, blend the ingredients for 45 seconds or until smooth and there are no visible pieces of fruit or nuts in the mixture.
3 tablespoons cashew or peanut butter	
1 tablespoon sesame seeds	**4** Pour the smoothie into 2 glasses and enjoy!

Per serving: Calories 421 (From Fat 175); Fat 19g (Saturated 6g); Cholesterol 22mg; Sodium 280mg; Carbohydrate 53g (Dietary Fiber 5g); Protein 15g.

Tip: Use one 6-ounce or two 4-ounce containers of raspberry or strawberry or other flavor fruit-on-the-bottom yogurt.

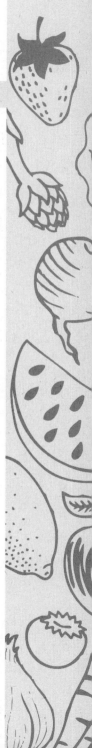

Orange Cow

Prep time: About 3 min • **Blending time:** 1 min • **Yield:** 2 servings

Ingredients	Directions
2 oranges 1 mango 1 cup fresh carrot juice 3 tablespoons powdered buttermilk	**1** Peel the oranges and break into sections. Remove the seeds.
	2 Peel the mango, remove the stone, and cut into chunks.
	3 Combine the carrot juice, oranges, mango, and buttermilk powder in the blender container.
	4 Secure the lid on the container.
	5 Starting on a low speed and gradually easing toward high, blend the ingredients for 45 seconds or until smooth and there are no visible pieces of fruit in the mixture.
	6 Pour the smoothie into 2 glasses and enjoy!

Per serving: Calories 200 (From Fat 11); Fat 1g (Saturated 1g); Cholesterol 8mg; Sodium 123mg; Carbohydrate 45g (Dietary Fiber 5g); Protein 7g.

Vary It! If you're juicing the carrots for this smoothie, try adding a parsnip or half a beet to vary the juice.

Tip: Taste the smoothie and add honey, maple syrup, or brown rice syrup if you want.

Berry Cheesy

Prep time: About 4 min • **Blending time:** 1 min • **Yield:** 2 servings

Ingredients	Directions
1 cup 1 percent or 2 percent milk	*1* Combine the milk and cottage cheese in the blender container.
¼ cup cottage cheese	
1 cup fresh or frozen strawberries	*2* Secure the lid on the container. Start blending on a low speed and gradually ease toward high, blending for 30 seconds.
¼ cup fresh or frozen blueberries	*3* Add strawberries, blueberries, and raspberries. If the berries are fresh, start blending on a low speed and gradually ease toward high, blending the ingredients for 45 seconds or until smooth and there are no visible pieces of fruit in the mixture.
¼ cup fresh or frozen raspberries	
	4 If the berries are frozen, start blending on a low speed and pulse for 30 seconds. Ease the speed toward high and blend the ingredients for 30 seconds or until smooth and there are no visible pieces of fruit in the mixture.
	5 Pour the smoothie into 2 glasses and enjoy!

Per serving: Calories 114 (From Fat 21); Fat 2g (Saturated 1g); Cholesterol 9mg; Sodium 162mg; Carbohydrate 17g (Dietary Fiber 3g); Protein 8g.

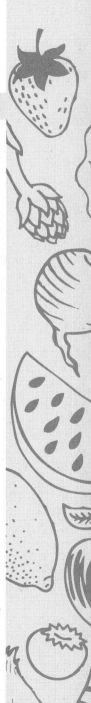

Breakfast Muesli

Prep time: About 4 min • **Blending time:** 1 min • **Yield:** 2 servings

Ingredients	Directions
1 cup 1 percent or 2 percent milk	**1** Combine the milk, yogurt, blueberries, oats, wheat germ, flaxseeds, sunflower seeds, and raisins in the blender container.
¼ cup plain 1 percent or 2 percent yogurt	
1 cup fresh or frozen blueberries	**2** Secure the lid on the container.
2 tablespoons rolled oats (large-flake or old-fashioned oatmeal)	**3** Starting on a low speed and gradually easing toward high, blend the ingredients for 45 seconds or until smooth and there are no visible pieces of fruit or nuts in the mixture.
2 tablespoons wheat germ	
1 tablespoon flaxseeds	**4** Pour the smoothie into 2 glasses and enjoy!
1 tablespoon sunflower seeds	

Per serving: Calories 203 (From Fat 61); Fat 7g (Saturated 2g); Cholesterol 7mg; Sodium 89mg; Carbohydrate 27g (Dietary Fiber 4g); Protein 11g.

Drinking at Midday: Lunch Smoothies

Using a dairy ingredient in smoothies for quick and nutritious lunchtime meals is an easy way to ensure that you're getting protein and calcium along with the vitamins and minerals from the milk products.

In addition to the liquid cow (or sheep or goat) milk, buttermilk, powdered milk, or evaporated milk listed earlier in this chapter, here are some other dairy products that work very well in lunch smoothies because their protein and fat stay with you throughout most of the afternoon:

- **Yogurt:** When milk is heated and beneficial bacteria are added, it ferments and becomes thickened and tart or lemony tasting. One cup of yogurt is higher in protein and calcium than an 8-ounce glass of liquid milk and it's easier to digest, so some lactose-intolerant people can eat it without problems.

- **Cheese:** Soft cheeses such as cottage, ricotta, mascarpone, creamy goat cheese, feta, and blue cheese may be spooned or crumbled into smoothies. Medium-hard cheese like cheddar, Swiss, and Gouda may be shredded for use in smoothies. Use 2 tablespoons of cheese for each smoothie serving.

- **Whey powder:** To make cheese, milk is heated and curdled so that solids form. The liquid left over from the curdled cheese solids is called *whey,* and it's dried and sold as a protein supplement. Adding 1 tablespoon of whey powder delivers about 15 grams of protein to a smoothie drink.

- **Cream:** Fresh, raw milk contains butterfat, which is light yellow and floats to the top. Supermarkets have various types of cream available and they differ only in the amount of butterfat they contain. Double cream has 48 percent butterfat; half-and-half cream has about 12 percent butterfat; and whipping cream (also called heavy cream) weighs in at 30 percent butterfat. Of course adding cream to smoothies makes them creamier and denser, but it's the fat that makes the drink so rich. For people who are undernourished and/or underweight, cream is an excellent addition to smoothies.

- **Crème fraîche:** In France, raw cream is thickened by bacteria for a slightly tangy, thick, and velvety smooth texture. Depending on the cream used to make it, crème fraîche may be as low as 20 percent or as high as 48 percent butterfat, so use it in smoothies with caution.

- **Sour cream:** Similar to crème fraîche, sour cream is fermented cream. By US law, the butterfat must be 18 percent or more, so reduced-fat sour cream is technically not sour cream. Commercial sour cream may contain gelatin, flavorings, vegetable enzymes, and sodium citrate.

Borscht

Prep time: About 4 min • **Blending time:** 1 min • **Cooking time:** 3–5 min • **Yield:** 2 servings

Ingredients	Directions
¾ cup fresh carrot juice	**1** Combine the carrot juice, yogurt, spinach, tomatoes, beets, and chopped dill in the blender container.
½ cup plain yogurt	
1 cup fresh spinach	**2** Secure the lid on the container.
2 tomatoes, peeled and quartered	**3** Starting on a low speed and gradually easing toward high, blend the ingredients for 45 seconds or until smooth and there are no visible pieces of vegetable in the mixture.
2 small, cooked beets, peeled and quartered	
2 teaspoons chopped fresh dill	**4** Pour into a saucepan and heat over medium-high heat for 3 to 5 minutes or until hot; or pour into a microwave-safe bowl and microwave on high for 1 minute or until hot.
2 sprigs fresh dill, for garnish (optional)	
	5 Pour the soup into 2 bowls, garnish with dill sprigs (if using), serve with a spoon, and enjoy!

Per serving: Calories 127 (From Fat 16); Fat 2g (Saturated 1g); Cholesterol 4mg; Sodium 179mg; Carbohydrate 24g (Dietary Fiber 4g); Protein 7g.

Tip: If you own a high-performance blender, skip Step 5 and run the machine at high for 4 to 6 minutes or until the soup is hot.

Vary It! Use ½ cup cottage cheese or ¼ cup sour cream in place of the yogurt if you want.

Creamy Tomato Soup

Prep time: About 3 min • **Blending time:** 1 min • **Cooking time:** 1–5 min • **Yield:** 2 servings

Ingredients	Directions
½ **cucumber**	*1* Peel the cucumber and cut it and the carrot into chunks.
1 carrot	
1 cup vegetable or chicken broth	*2* Combine the broth, tomatoes, yogurt, kale, cilantro, cucumber, and carrot in the blender container.
4 tomatoes, quartered	
½ **cup drained yogurt or Greek-style yogurt**	*3* Secure the lid on the container.
1 cup chopped kale or Swiss chard	*4* Starting on a low speed and gradually easing toward high, blend the ingredients for 45 seconds or until smooth and there are no visible pieces of vegetable in the mixture.
¼ **cup cilantro or parsley**	
	5 Pour the soup into a saucepan and heat over medium heat, stirring constantly for 5 to 10 minutes or until hot; or pour into a microwave-safe bowl and microwave on high for 1 minute or until hot.
	6 Pour the soup into 2 bowls, serve with a spoon, and enjoy!

Per serving: *Calories 160 (From Fat 25); Fat 3g (Saturated 1g); Cholesterol 4mg; Sodium 589mg; Carbohydrate 29g (Dietary Fiber 4g); Protein 8g.*

Tip: If you own high-performance blender, skip Step 5 and run the machine at high for 4 to 6 minutes or until the soup is hot.

Tip: Stir constantly while heating to keep yogurt from curdling.

Vary It! You can garnish the soup with a tablespoon of drained yogurt if you want.

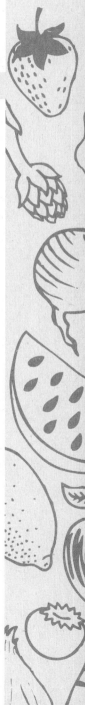

Chicken Salad

Prep time: About 4 min • **Blending time:** 1 min • **Yield:** 2 servings

Ingredients	Directions
1 cup chicken broth	**1** Combine the broth, spinach, cabbage, carrot, whey powder, and sunflower seeds in the blender container.
2 cups fresh or chopped frozen spinach	
1 cup coarsely chopped cabbage	**2** Secure the lid on the container.
1 carrot	**3** Starting on a low speed and gradually easing toward high, blend the ingredients for 45 seconds or until smooth and there are no visible pieces of vegetable in the mixture.
2 tablespoons whey powder	
1 tablespoon sunflower seeds	
1 cup shredded, cooked chicken	**4** Add the chicken to the container and pulse for 10 to 20 seconds or until just mixed in but still in pieces.
	5 Pour the smoothie into 2 glasses, serve with a spoon, and enjoy!

Per serving: Calories 227 (From Fat 62); Fat 7g (Saturated 2g); Cholesterol 62mg; Sodium 664mg; Carbohydrate 10g (Dietary Fiber 3g); Protein 30g.

Mixing Up Some Dairy Mocktail and Cocktail Smoothies

Why dairy cocktails and nonalcoholic drinks, you might ask? First, because they're delicious — think Bailey's and Kahlúa — and they supply protein and calcium for added nutrients. However, as with most cocktail drinks, the calories are stacked pretty high when these drinks are compared to plain vegetable or even fruit smoothies.

The same amount of smoothie ingredients that serves two in the fruit and vegetable section is suggested to serve four here. Serve them in shot glasses and sip slowly if you want to lower the calories you consume with each drink. Of course, if you drink twice as many because they're just so darned tasty, this defeats that strategy.

I suggest a darker alcohol such as amber rum, rye, or Scotch, instead of lighter spirits because the cream mixer can take the stronger tasting liquor. If you prefer a lighter taste, of course, you can use vodka, light rum, or gin. Liqueurs make good additions to smoothies, and I use an orange-flavored one in the Orange Cream recipe here. Table 18-1 provides a brief list of some liqueurs that add other flavors you can experiment with in smoothies.

Table18-1	Some Liqueurs to Add to Dairy Smoothies
Liqueur	*Flavor*
Crème de cassis	Black currant
Chambord	Raspberry
Anisette, Anis, Cartujo	Anise flavor (licorice)
Kahlúa, Tia Maria, Café Aztec, Bahia	Coffee
Advocaat	Cream and eggs
Dulce de Leche	Caramel and cream
Heather Cream	Scotch and cream
St-Germain	Elderflower
Cointreau, Curacao, Grand Marnier	Orange
PAMA, DeKuyper Pomegranate	Pomegranate

Crème Cassis

Prep time: About 3 min • **Blending time:** 1 min • **Yield:** 4 servings

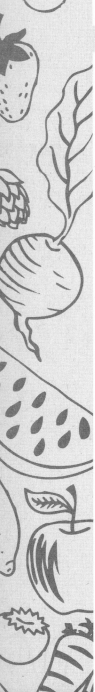

Ingredients	Directions
1 cup 18 percent to 35 percent cream	*1* Combine the cream, yogurt, ice cream, blackberries, and cocoa in the blender container.
½ cup vanilla yogurt	
1 scoop vanilla ice cream	*2* Secure the lid on the container.
2 cups fresh or frozen blackberries	*3* Starting on a low speed and gradually easing toward high, blend the ingredients for 45 seconds or until smooth and there are no visible pieces of fruit in the mixture.
2 teaspoons dark chocolate cocoa, optional	
4 ounces amber rum	*4* Pour the drink into 4 glasses, stir 1 ounce of alcohol into each drink, and enjoy!

Per serving: Calories 353 (From Fat 213); Fat 24g (Saturated 15g); Cholesterol 87mg; Sodium 50mg; Carbohydrate 18g (Dietary Fiber 4g); Protein 4g.

Vary It! Frozen fruit makes a smoothie thicker. You can use any frozen berry in place of the blackberries. Raspberries, blueberries, and strawberries work, as do other pieces of frozen fruit, so experiment.

Café au Lait

Prep time: About 4 min • **Blending time:** 1 min • **Yield:** 4 servings

Ingredients	Directions
½ cup whole milk or 10 percent cream	**1** Combine the milk or cream, yogurt, ice cream, coffee beans, and melted chocolate in the blender container.
1 cup plain yogurt	
1 scoop chocolate ice cream	**2** Secure the lid on the container.
¼ cup chocolate-covered coffee beans	**3** Starting on a low speed and gradually easing toward high, blend the ingredients for 45 seconds or until smooth and there are no visible pieces of the beans in the mixture.
2 tablespoons melted dark chocolate	
	4 Pour the mocktail into 4 glasses and enjoy!

Per serving: Calories 149 (From Fat 68); Fat 8g (Saturated 5g); Cholesterol 11mg; Sodium 65mg; Carbohydrate 17g (Dietary Fiber 1g); Protein 5g.

Vary It! You can use chocolate syrup in place of the melted chocolate.

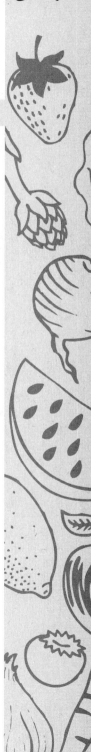

Crème de Banane

Prep time: About 4 min • **Blending time:** 1 min • **Yield:** 4 servings

Ingredients	Directions
1 cup buttermilk	**1** Combine the buttermilk, yogurt, banana, ice cream, cinnamon, and nutmeg in the blender container.
½ cup plain yogurt	
4 chunks frozen banana	**2** Secure the lid on the container.
1 scoop vanilla ice cream	
⅛ teaspoon ground cinnamon	**3** Starting on a low speed and gradually easing toward high, blend the ingredients for 45 seconds or until smooth and there are no visible pieces of fruit in the mixture.
⅛ teaspoon ground nutmeg	
	4 Pour the mocktail into 4 glasses and enjoy!

Per serving: Calories 88 (From Fat 19); Fat 2g (Saturated 1g); Cholesterol 8mg; Sodium 93mg; Carbohydrate 14g (Dietary Fiber 1g); Protein 4g.

Tip: You can use one fresh banana cut into chunks in place of the frozen banana.

Orange Cream

Prep time: About 4 min • **Blending time:** 1 min • **Yield:** 4 servings

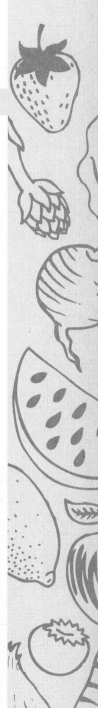

Ingredients	Directions
1 orange **1 cup half and half (10 percent) or light (18 percent) cream** **½ cup vanilla yogurt** **1 tablespoon grated orange rind** **1 scoop vanilla ice cream** **2 ounces orange flavored liqueur**	*1* Grate 1 tablespoon of orange peel and set aside in a small bowl. Peel and seed the orange and break it into quarters. *2* Combine the milk, yogurt, grated rind, orange sections, and ice cream in the blender container. *3* Secure the lid on the container. *4* Starting on a low speed and gradually easing toward high, blend the ingredients for 45 seconds or until smooth and there are no visible pieces of fruit in the mixture. *5* Pour the drink into 4 glasses, stir ½ ounce of liqueur into each drink, and enjoy!

Per serving: Calories 227 (From Fat 114); Fat 13g (Saturated 8g); Cholesterol 44mg; Sodium 51mg; Carbohydrate 20g (Dietary Fiber 1g); Protein 4g.

Feed your curiosity

You love fruit. (Who doesn't?) You can't resist the clear zing of flavors that seem to burst with sweet vitality. So, it's likely that you have your favorites — the old standbys that you gravitate toward in the produce section again and again.

Chances are, if you keep choosing the same fruit and vegetables for juices and smoothies, as great as they are, you're always getting the same phytonutrients and missing out on all the other good things that are part of the wide spectrum available. To get the most out of your juices and smoothies and put the finest into your body, you need to include some of each of all the colors — red, green, orange, and blue — every day. And I'm not just talking about fruit. Vegetables have so much to offer (I list the specific nutrients in Chapter 6).

My advice is to get curious about how the taste of something you love will blend with something you hardly ever eat. Because juices and smoothies are a purée — a mixture of tastes and textures — every day you get to be a bit of an alchemist, mingling, melding, integrating, and designing your own amalgam of perfection!

Chapter 19

Focusing on After Dinner: Frozen Smoothies

In this chapter, you explore the convenient and easy ways to delight and refresh yourself with frozen smoothies. Most of these recipes are light and only have a few ingredients, so they're simple to make.

Eat frozen smoothies immediately after you make them — you don't need to freeze and stir and refreeze them.

If the fruit or liquid you're using is tart, you can sweeten it with 1 or 2 table-spoons of maple or brown rice syrup, sugar, or honey (or to taste).

Making Frozen Treats

If you have a high-performance machine or a powerful blender with either variable speeds or a pulse function, you can make ice-cold refreshing drinks with textures that range from spoon-able to very thin and pourable. The only difference is in the amount of ice and frozen fruit you use. Table 19-1 pro-vides a general guide to four types of frozen treats and drinks that will allow you to use a wide variety of flavors, tailoring them to your own taste.

Freezing smoothies in advance

Even with the incredible ease of making smoothies, some morning-challenged people love the option of making a large batch of healthy smoothies on the weekend or when convenient. Thawed overnight in the refrigerator, they make a quick quencher on weekday mornings.

To make freezer smoothies for weekday breakfasts, choose any of the pure fruit or vegetable smoothie recipes in Chapters 16 or 17, and omit alcohol and high-calorie ingredients. *Note:* Some people don't like the texture of frozen smoothies containing milk, cheese, or yogurt, so you'll have to experiment with those recipes to determine your preferences.

Once you've chosen your recipe, follow these steps:

1. **Make a single or double smoothie recipe of your choice.**
2. **Divide the smoothie evenly and pour it into small zip-top freezer bags (one bag per serving).**
3. **Label each bag with the recipe name and date, and store in the freezer for up to three months.**
4. **Remove a bag from the freezer the night before you want to drink it, and thaw it in the refrigerator for use in the morning.**
5. **In the morning, pour the smoothie into a glass or open the bag enough to thrust a straw into the smoothie and go!**

Table 19-1	Four Types of Frozen Smoothies		
Type of Smoothie	*Amount of Liquid*	*Amount of Frozen Berries or Fruit Pieces*	*Amount of Ice*
Very thick or spoonable	1 cup	2 cups	1 cup
Thick	1½ cups	1½ cups	1 cup
Thin	2 cups	1½ cups	½ cup
Very thin or pourable	2 cups	1 cup	½ cup

Chilling with Iced Smoothies

The drinks in this section are inspired by the Italian iced treat called *gelato*. Strictly speaking, gelato is a frozen custard or blend of whole milk, sugar, and egg yolks that has been heated until the proteins in the milk and egg yolks thicken it. A wide range of flavoring ingredients (from chocolate or coffee to fresh berries to herbs and spices) is added and the custard is chilled and stirred to incorporate air for a velvety smooth and rich-tasting result. Gelato is similar to but denser than ice cream because less air is incorporated into the custard base.

They aren't truly healthy — even with the fresh fruit — but how can you resist these sugary, creamy treats? The answer is to blend your own gelato-inspired smoothies with less sugar (and other sweeteners) and without using cream or egg yolks.

You can use any type of liquid milk in these smoothies: whole, 2 percent, 1 percent, or skim milk; buttermilk; or sheep or goat milk.

Clean the machine first

One rule my husband and I always observe (and insisted that our daughter follow as well) is that we never even taste the drink before the machine is cleaned. It worked for our family, and we never returned to the kitchen to find a sticky mess.

To clean a blender, follow these steps:

1. **Splash a couple drops of liquid soap (no more!) into the container.**

2. **Add hot water straight from the tap, filling it up to about the middle of the container.**

3. **Place the lid on it and blend, starting on low and moving to medium, for 3 seconds.**

The hot, soapy water is enough to clean the blades and the sides of the container.

4. **Remove the lid, pour the soapy water over the inside of the lid, rinse the lid and the container.**

5. **Wipe the motor (be sure the machine is unplugged first), and set the container in position for the next time. Some people like to turn the container and lid upside down on a dish rack or a clean tea towel to dry.**

Walnut and Mascarpone Ice

Prep time: About 2 min • **Blending time:** 1 min • **Yield:** 2 servings

Ingredients	Directions
1 cup low-fat milk	*1* Combine the milk, vanilla, and honey in the blender container.
1 teaspoon pure vanilla extract	
1 to 4 tablespoons honey, to taste	*2* Secure the lid on the container.
½ cup (4 ounces) mascarpone cheese	*3* Starting on a low speed and gradually easing toward high, blend the ingredients for 20 seconds or until smooth.
½ cup chopped walnuts	
1 cup ice cubes	*4* Add the mascarpone and blend on medium speed for 30 seconds or until blended into the milk mixture. Add walnuts and blend on medium speed for 30 seconds or until there are no visible pieces of walnuts in the mixture.
	5 Add ice and starting on a low speed, gradually ease toward high and blend for 30 seconds or until the ice is mixed into the mixture and it is smooth. If you have a tamping stick, use it to move the ice around; otherwise, you may need to stop and stir the mixture, freeing the ice around the blades, and resume blending. (If you're using a blender with a pulse button, pulse the blades on and off until the ice is chopped and the mixture is smooth.)
	6 Spoon the ice into 2 glasses, serve with a spoon, and enjoy!

Per serving: Calories 535 (From Fat 425); Fat 47g (Saturated 17g); Cholesterol 78mg; Sodium 97mg; Carbohydrate 21g; Dietary Fiber 2g; Protein 13g.

Vary It! You can use cottage cheese in place of the mascarpone cheese if you prefer.

Vary It! You can substitute pecans or hazelnuts for the walnuts.

Mocha Ice

Prep time: About 2 min • **Blending time:** 1 minute • **Yield:** 2 servings

Ingredients	Directions
1 cup 10 percent to 18 percent cream	***1*** Combine the cream, coffee, vanilla, and ice cream in the blender container.
¼ cup espresso coffee, chilled	
1 teaspoon pure vanilla extract	***2*** Secure the lid on the container.
1 scoop chocolate ice cream (about ½ cup)	***3*** Starting on a low speed and gradually easing toward high, blend the ingredients for 30 seconds or until smooth.
2 tablespoons chopped bittersweet chocolate, melted	
1 cup ice cubes	***4*** With blender running on a medium speed, add melted chocolate through the opening in the lid. Blend for 15 seconds or until well mixed. Add ice and start blending on a low speed. Gradually increase to high and blend for 35 seconds or until smooth. If you have a tamping stick, use it to move the ice around; otherwise, you may need to stop and stir the mixture, freeing the ice around the blades, and resume blending. (If you're using a blender with a pulse button, pulse the blades on and off until the ice is chopped and the mixture is smooth.)
	5 Spoon the ice into 2 glasses, serve with a spoon, and enjoy!

Per serving: Calories 326 (From Fat 214); Fat 24g (Saturated 15g); Cholesterol 51mg; Sodium 63mg; Carbohydrate 25g; Dietary Fiber 2g; Protein 5g.

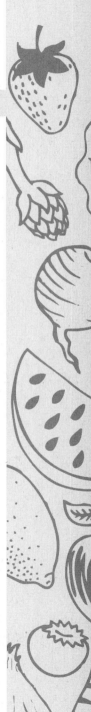

Adding Shaved Ice: Granite

The word *granite* gives you an indication of the texture of these iced treats. Similar to the chipped or shaved ice drizzled with flavored syrup and served in paper cones or cups you may have enjoyed at amusement parks when you were a kid, granite are the simplest of all frozen desserts.

The dessert version of this chilled treat is made from fruit and sugar that is cooked or puréed, spread into shallow pans, frozen, and stirred frequently to keep it from freezing into a solid block of ice. When ice forming in the fruit-sugar mixture is stirred, it gets broken into smaller pieces that ultimately cause the granita's texture to resemble sand or granite. The more sugar used, the easier it is to keep the granita from forming a solid frozen brick.

My blended versions use the same fruit and sugar combinations, but the addition of ice to the blender makes them ready to consume instantly.

The singular form of *granite* is *granita*.

Easy frozen granite

For an easy method of achieving the Italian ices popular on the streets of Italian (and some North American) cities in the summer, double the amount of liquid, fruit, and sugar in either of the recipes in this section. Omit the ice and use fresh fruit instead of frozen fruit. Blend until smooth, pour the mixture into one or two ice-cube trays, and freeze for at least three hours and up to two days in advance.

Note: Place the ice-cube tray in the coldest part of the freezer. In a chest freezer, the coldest place is the floor, while in an upright freezer, that spot is usually at the top of the freezer. Allow some space around the trays for cold air to circulate — this will help the mixture to freeze quicker.

Unmold the cubes into the blender container and secure the lid. Starting on a low speed and gradually easing toward high, blend the ingredients for 45 seconds or until smooth and there are no visible pieces of fruit in the mixture. If you have a tamping stick, use it to move the cubes around; otherwise, you may need to stop and stir the mixture, freeing the frozen purée around the blades, and resume blending. (If you're using a blender with a pulse button, pulse the blades on and off just until the cubes are chopped and the mixture is smooth.)

Granite made this way will be stronger in taste because the ice, which tends to dilute the taste, has not been added to them.

Lemon Granita

Prep time: About 2 min • **Blending time:** 1 min • **Yield:** 2 servings

Ingredients	Directions
1 tablespoon lemon rind	**1** Grate the 1 tablespoon of lemon rind into the blender container.
1 lemon	
½ cup fresh orange juice	**2** Peel the lemon, break into sections, and remove the seeds.
½ cup fresh lemon juice	
½ to 1 cup sugar, to taste	**3** Combine the orange juice, lemon juice, and sugar in the blender container. Taste and add more sugar if needed. Add lemon, lemon rind, and ice.
1 cup ice cubes	
	4 Secure the lid on the container.
	5 Starting on a low speed and gradually easing toward high, blend the ingredients for 45 seconds or until smooth and there are no visible pieces of fruit in the mixture. If you have a tamping stick, use it to move the ice around; otherwise, you may need to stop and stir the mixture, freeing the fruit and ice around the blades, and resume blending. (If you're using a blender with a pulse button, pulse the blades on and off until the ice is chopped and the mixture is smooth.)
	6 Spoon the granita into 2 martini or wine glasses, serve with a spoon, and enjoy!

Per serving: Calories 244 (From Fat 1); Fat 0g (Saturated 0g); Cholesterol 0mg; Sodium 4mg; Carbohydrate 64g; Dietary Fiber 1g; Protein 1g.

Vary It! To make this drink icier, pour the mixture into a shallow pan and freeze for up to 40 minutes. Scrape the ice into 2 glasses and serve with a spoon.

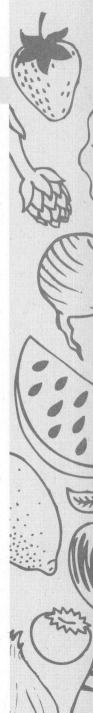

Mango Granita

Prep time: About 2 min • **Blending time:** 1 min • **Yield:** 2 servings

Ingredients	Directions
3 mangoes	*1* Peel the mangoes, cut them in half, and remove the flat stone.
½ cup fresh orange juice	
½ cup fresh apricot nectar	*2* Combine the orange juice, apricot nectar, lemon juice, and sugar in the blender container.
1 tablespoon lemon juice	
½ to 1 cup sugar, to taste	*3* Secure the lid on the container.
1 cup ice cubes	
	4 Starting on a low speed and gradually easing toward high, blend the ingredients for 15 seconds or until sugar is dissolved into juice. Taste and add more sugar if needed.
	5 Add mangoes and ice. Start blending on a low speed and increase to high. Blend for 30 seconds or until smooth. If you have a tamping stick, use it to move the ice around; otherwise, you may need to stop and stir the mixture, freeing the fruit and ice around the blades, and resume blending. (If you're using a blender with a pulse button, pulse the blades on and off until the ice is chopped and the mixture is smooth.)
	6 Spoon the granita into 2 martini or wine glasses, serve with a spoon, and enjoy!

Per serving: Calories 460 (From Fat 9); Fat 1g (Saturated 0g); Cholesterol 0mg; Sodium 9mg; Carbohydrate 119g; Dietary Fiber 6g; Protein 2g.

Vary It! You can use grapefruit juice or orange juice in place of the apricot nectar.

Vary It! To make this drink icier, pour the mixture into a shallow pan and freeze for up to 40 minutes. Scrape the ice into 2 glasses, and serve with a spoon.

Serving Some Sherbets and Sorbets

Elizabeth David gives an interesting account of the history of ice and ice desserts in her book, *Harvest of the Cold Months: The Social History of Ice and Ices* (Penguin Books). Using interesting stories and tales of ancient uses for snow and ice, David explains how ice was harvested, transported, and stored for the dinner tables of the urban upper class. Her account of neiges (snow), sorbets, glaces, and ices are entertaining and insightful.

Derived from *sharbāt,* the Arabic word for fruit syrup, our modern sherbet is descended from those refreshing luxuries of fruit syrup or condensed juices drizzled over snow. What most likely began as an indulgent treat exclusively for royalty has become a favorite of many Westerners.

Somewhere in the long journey from the deserts of the Middle East to Europe and subsequently to North America, sherbets became infused with dairy — sometimes milk only, sometimes milk and eggs — to the point where an actual definition is difficult to achieve. In simplified terms, our modern sherbet is a mixture of milk or cream, sugar, and some flavoring.

To confuse the issue further, what used to be called *ice milk* in the United States, was actually a milk sherbet. Today, due to regulatory changes by the US Department of Agriculture (USDA), that product is called *low-fat ice cream.*

Sorbet is a non-dairy frozen product that contains only fruit, sugar, and some flavoring along with gelatin for stabilizing the frozen product.

Both sherbets and sorbet are best when eaten soft and served in small bowls, martini glasses, or ice cream sundae cups. Often served between courses, sherbet or sorbet serves to cleanse the palate for the next course.

Raspberry Sherbet

Prep time: About 2 min • **Blending time:** 1 min • **Yield:** 2 servings

Ingredients	Directions
1 cup low-fat milk	*1* Combine the milk, juice, honey, raspberries, and ice in the blender container.
¼ cup pomegranate or grape juice	
1 to 4 tablespoons honey, to taste	*2* Secure the lid on the container.
2 cups frozen raspberries	*3* Starting on a low speed and gradually easing toward high, blend the ingredients for 45 seconds or until smooth and there are no visible pieces of fruit in the mixture. If you have a tamping stick, use it to move the ice around; otherwise, you may need to stop and stir the mixture, freeing the fruit and ice around the blades, and resume blending.
1 cup ice cubes	
	4 Spoon the sherbet into 2 glasses, serve with a spoon, and enjoy!

Per serving: Calories 164 (From Fat 18); Fat 2g (Saturated 1g); Cholesterol 5mg; Sodium 64mg; Carbohydrate 34g; Dietary Fiber 8g; Protein 5g.

Tip: To determine the amount of sweetener to use, taste the smoothie and add honey or maple syrup or brown rice syrup by the tablespoon until you reach the desired sweetness.

Citrus Sorbet

Prep time: About 2 min • **Blending time:** 1 min • **Yield:** 2 servings

Ingredients	Directions
1 cup orange juice	*1* Combine the juice, honey, frozen concentrate, frozen orange or grapefruit sections, and ice in the blender container.
1 to 4 tablespoons honey, to taste	
¼ cup frozen lemon or lime concentrate	*2* Secure the lid on the container.
2 cups frozen orange or grapefruit sections	*3* Starting on a low speed and gradually easing toward high, blend the ingredients for 45 seconds or until smooth and there are no visible pieces of fruit in the mixture. If you have a tamping stick, use it to move the ice around; otherwise, you may need to stop and stir the mixture, freeing the fruit and ice around the blades, and resume blending.
1 cup ice cubes	
	4 Spoon the sorbet into 2 glasses, serve with a spoon, and enjoy!

Per serving: Calories 239 (From Fat 5); Fat 1g (Saturated 0g); Cholesterol 0mg; Sodium 3mg; Carbohydrate 60g; Dietary Fiber 5g; Protein 3g.

Vary It! You can use frozen blueberries or other fruit in place of the orange or grapefruit sections.

Tip: To freeze orange or grapefruit sections, peel, section, and seed them. Arrange in a single layer on a parchment-lined baking sheet, and freeze for at least an hour. If not using right away, transfer to a freezer bag, seal and label it, and store in the freezer for up to 3 months.

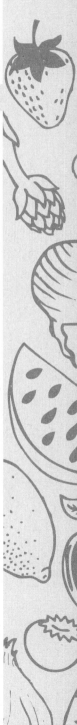

Make 'em thick

One of the outstanding characteristics of smoothies — after their creamy texture, of course — is their thick consistency. Some of that thickness comes from the fiber and cellulose in the fruits and vegetables. That banana in the very first smoothie ever made was there not just because of its pretty taste. In fact, banana is used in smoothies as the prime thickener.

Here are some ingredients to use to replace banana in smoothies and still get that thick consistency. Add them directly to the blender with all the other ingredients in place of the banana:

- ½ sliced avocado

- ¼ cup drained yogurt

- ¼ cup old-fashioned rolled oats (large flake oatmeal)

- 2 tablespoons chia seeds, soaked in ¼ cup water for 10 minutes or finely ground and added directly to smoothie ingredients

- ¼ cup silken tofu

Another way to blend really thick smoothies is to add ice or frozen fruits or vegetables. I prefer to add frozen produce, but ice is a good choice for people who want to control their weight, because it has the added bonus of being completely free of calories, sugar, and fat.

Coconut water is becoming widely available, and it makes a refreshingly tasty liquid for smoothies. It must be stored in the refrigerator and used within five days. If you don't use all the coconut water before the end of the recommended storage time, it can be frozen in ice cube trays and added to smoothies in the same way as ice is added. You also can freeze fresh juice in exactly the same way.

Part V
The Part of Tens

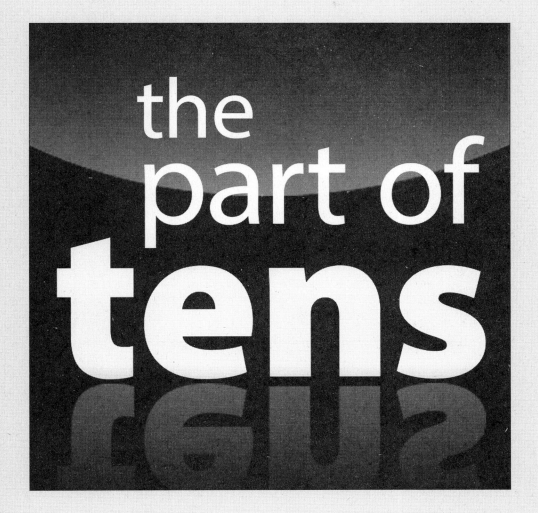

Refer to www.dummies.com/extras/juicingsmoothies for a ten common questions often asked about juicing and smoothies.

In this part . . .

- ✔ Identify the best antioxidant-rich and immune-building fruits and vegetables to use in juices and smoothies.

- ✔ Understand how antioxidants attack free radicals and help your body to operate more like it naturally should.

- ✔ Investigate the benefits of immune-building nutrients to your health so that you can defend yourself against common ailments.

Chapter 20

Ten Antioxidant-Rich Fruits and Vegetables

In This Chapter

▶ Understanding how antioxidants work

▶ Using high-powered antioxidants for optimum results

▶ Preventing degenerative diseases

*E*veryone is rusting on the inside. Yup, you read that right. You and I are oxidizing, which is the same thing that happens when air attacks metal and causes it to corrode or rust. Ever left a cut apple out on the counter? If not, try it and see how fast it turns brown. The oxygen in the air is attacking or rusting the cells in the apple that are exposed. The same thing happens to your cells and organs and causes serious damage, leading to aging and degenerative diseases.

Free radicals are unstable oxygen molecules caused by stress, chemicals, pollutants, toxins and just plain living. They attack your cells in order to steal extra electrons and, in the process, cause healthy, normal cells to die, mutate, or become weak and susceptible to disease.

Antioxidants found in plant foods stop free radicals from doing their damage, but you have to eat enough of them in order for them to work their magic. Remember that cut apple? Try brushing lemon juice on a freshly cut apple and wait for it to turn brown. It won't, because the vitamin C in the lemon juice is an antioxidant that protects the flesh from being attacked by oxygen. The best antioxidants are found in the pigments that give plants their color. In this chapter, I list the very best antioxidant fruit and vegetables. Choose one or two from this list to use as an ingredient in a smoothie or juice or eat them fresh in salads or as a snack — just be sure to get lots of them every single day!

Refer to www.dummies.com/extras/juicingsmoothies for how you can measure antioxidant value.

Acai Berries

The acai palm grows in the Amazon rain forest of Brazil. Its berries, called acai (pronounced *ah*-sigh-*ee*) are large and plump, about the size of a grape. What's amazing about them is their dark blue-purple color and their taste, which is somewhere between a blueberry and chocolate.

Although Brazilians have enjoyed acai berries as a fresh fruit for hundreds of years, they have just recently been growing in popularity in North America. The fresh berry is not widely available, but the frozen fruit and the juice (as well as a powder made from the juice) are available in health food stores.

Black Raspberries

Commonly called blackcaps, these native North American berries are currently being grown commercially in the Pacific Northwest. Although the fresh berries are available only for a very short time, the frozen and dried powdered fruit is more widely distributed.

Eat the seeds, too! Using fresh or frozen whole blackcaps in smoothies is especially healthy because the oil in raspberry seeds is rich in vitamin E and omega-3 fatty acids.

Wild Blueberries and Cranberries

No doubt about it, cultivated blueberries are very good for you, but wild blueberries score over twice as high in antioxidants. They're available in the Northeast during midsummer and frozen at other times of the year.

Raw cranberries are a native of North America and are widely available fresh in the late fall and frozen throughout the year. They make an excellent fresh juice if teamed with sweeter fruits such as apples or pineapples. Fresh or frozen cranberries are a good choice as an ingredient for smoothies, but you may need some sweetener because the flavor is very tart. The whole berries are best, but the unsweetened juice is moderately high in antioxidants, too.

Black Plums and Prunes

Black plums are high in vitamins C, K, and A, as well as fiber and antioxidants. Use pitted fresh black plums in juices and fresh or frozen in smoothies.

Prunes, which are the dried version of a European plum, are incredibly high in fiber, which is beneficial in reducing the risk of colorectal cancer. It's the phenolic compounds in both plums and prunes that make them high in antioxidants. Use pitted prunes in smoothies.

Blackberries

There's a pattern here — can you see it? All five of the high-antioxidant fruits are very dark: purple, blue, or black. It's the powerful antioxidant pigments in the skin and flesh that score high. Not surprisingly, blackberries are a very good addition to smoothies and excellent in fresh juices.

Red Beans, Kidney Beans, and Black Beans

Many legumes — specifically, black turtle beans, soybeans, red kidney beans, pinto beans, black-eyed peas, and lentils — score high in antioxidants, but only in their *raw* state. Once you boil them, their antioxidant scores drop by roughly one-third.

For smoothies and juices, if you have a powerful blender (like a high-performance blender; see Chapter 3), you can grind your own dried beans or lentils or you can buy ground or powdered beans or bean flour in specialty food stores.

Artichokes

I know, they're hard to clean and cook, but the antioxidant power of artichokes is high enough for them to make this list, and you can purchase them cooked and preserved in water. Use artichoke hearts as an ingredient in smoothies, not only for their antioxidant properties, but also because they stimulate the production of bile in the liver, help gallbladder functioning, and reduce cholesterol.

Garlic

You might think of garlic strictly as an herb, something to add flavor to dishes. I recommend that you use it as a vegetable and in quantities that can positively affect your health.

Although you'll likely be able to tolerate only one-half raw clove to one whole raw clove of garlic in vegetable drinks, including it will help to boost your overall daily consumption, which should be two to four cloves a day (or about one whole head of garlic per week) for the best medical benefits.

Cabbage and Broccoli Rabe

Both cabbage and broccoli rabe are high in phytonutrients. Red cabbage contains 36 different varieties of *anthocyanins,* those powerful antioxidants found in the black, purple, blue, and red plant pigments. Use it in juicing and smoothies for its calcium; magnesium; potassium; and vitamins C, K, and A. One cup of cooked cabbage supplies 4 grams of fiber, so lightly steam or simmer it for use in smoothies.

Broccoli rabe is a bitter-tasting relative of broccoli, with more leaves and a smaller flower head. Although broccoli is very good and shouldn't be ignored, broccoli rabe scores as high as red cabbage as an antioxidant and like its plumper, less bitter cousin, it's low in calories and high in calcium, potassium, vitamin C, folate, and vitamins K and A. Use broccoli rabe raw in juicing and either raw or lightly steamed in smoothies.

Purple Cauliflower

Like purple and white carrots, purple cauliflower is making its way into farmers' markets and onto supermarket shelves. Both white and purple cauliflower are rich in *sulforaphane,* a powerful antioxidant. If you can't find the purple variety, eat the yellow or the white, but eat it two or three times a week because it helps to neutralize and rid your cells of carcinogenic molecules. One cup of raw cauliflower provides 85 percent of your daily vitamin C requirements; it also supplies vitamin K, folate, choline, vitamin B6, potassium, fiber, and manganese, among other nutrients.

Chapter 21

Ten Immune-Building Ingredients

*E*ver wonder why some people sail through cold and flu season unscathed? Others travel often, work late, and still get through stressful times without a cough or sniffle? You're only as strong as your body's defense system, and making sure that it's running at peak performance should be one of your first health priorities. This chapter gives you ten dietary tips to building a strong immune system and keeping its complex cells functioning to protect your body against infection and disease.

Front-line defense tactics include adequate sleep and exercise, stress reduction, and frequent hand washing. Consuming immune-building and antioxidant foods is also vital for protecting against all sorts of pathogenic organisms that may enter and harm your body, for destroying cancerous cells, and for speeding healing from injury and infections. Foods rich in vitamins A, B complex, C, E, and K; choline, zinc, iron, copper, selenium, and manganese; as well as essential fatty acids and fiber are essential to a healthy immune system. You can find them all in a wide range of fruits and vegetables, whole grains, herbs, legumes, nuts, seeds, and small amounts of shellfish, cold-water fish, and extra-virgin olive oil.

It's no coincidence that the very same foods that neutralize free radicals, preventing them from damaging cells, are also high on the list of those that help prevent degenerative diseases. This is because after cells are mutated or weakened by free radicals, aging processes and diseases can gain a foothold. By disarming rampaging free radicals, antioxidants virtually escort them out of the body.

With uncompromised and healthy cells, the mucus membranes in your nose, throat, and other parts of your immune system can function at optimum efficiency, and you're better able to withstand inevitable virus invasions. Here is a simplified explanation of how viruses work their black magic. All viruses have spikes that puncture cells at weak spots and infect them, causing you to sniffle, cough, and react with other various symptoms in different areas of your body.

Use this chapter to discover about the top ten juice and smoothie ingredients for boosting immunity that may be main ingredients or easily added to smoothies and juices.

Antioxidant Black Fruits

All antioxidants, especially black fruits, such as black plums and blackberries, are powerful tools that work to protect your cells from damage so that viruses can't find an easy way to infect cells. Refer to Chapter 20 for a list of antioxidant black fruits and vegetables to include in immune-building smoothies and juices.

Cranberries for Urinary Tract Protection

Researchers have found that cranberries (and other berries such as lingonberries) contain substances that keep bacteria from sticking to the walls of the urinary tract. Researchers aren't certain whether antioxidants in the cranberries actually disarm or slime the hooks on the bacteria or if cranberries actually coat the urinary tract. Either way, with the intervention of cranberries, severely impaired bacteria can't get a grip and infect the urinary tract.

Fresh, whole cranberries are available in the fall. You can find frozen whole berries at most supermarkets all year round. Use them with antioxidant fruits and vegetables in juice and smoothies around cold and flu season or at the change of the seasons.

Should you experience burning or bladder pain, take four to six glasses of cranberry juice immediately throughout the first day. See your healthcare provider if the symptoms persist.

Red and Purple Grapes

The immune-building and antioxidant protector in red and purple (also called Concord) grapes is *resveratrol*, which has been shown to have the ability to protect your body from radiation and your skin from skin cancer. As an anti-inflammatory, resveratrol is effective in helping blood to flow more easily through blood vessels, thus lowering the risk of heart disease. It also may lower blood sugar levels as much as 10 percent.

British researchers found that resveratrol increases blood flow to the brain, leading them to conclude that resveratrol may help speed mental responses. Swiss tests proved that resveratrol is able to clear plaques and free radicals from the brain, two critical substances linked to Alzheimer's disease.

 Due to the powerful antioxidant pigments in the skin of red and purple grapes, adding them whole to smoothies gives you an edge over juicing them and having the skins separated out.

Cruciferous Vegetables

Broccoli, cauliflower, kale, Brussels sprouts, bok choy, rutabaga, turnips, and cabbage are part of a family of vegetables called *cruciferous* because their tiny flowers form a cross. All are high in vitamins A, C, E and K, folate, and minerals. They're powerful antioxidants and offer a good source of fiber.

 In addition, cruciferous vegetables contain chemicals called *glucosinolates,* which give them their strong flavor and aroma. These substances have been found to inhibit the development of cancer by protecting cells from DNA damage and by helping to inactivate carcinogens. They have both antibacterial and anti-inflammatory effects, and they're excellent antioxidant

 Juicing fresh, raw cruciferous vegetables is easy. Although you can add them raw to smoothies, you may want to lightly steam them first to tame their flavors and make them easy to blend, especially if you don't have a high-performance machine.

Shiitake Mushrooms

Known as a symbol of longevity in Asia, shiitake mushrooms offer support to the immune system when needed. New studies have revealed their ability to protect against rheumatoid arthritis and also help protect heart health by lowering cholesterol and keeping blood vessels clear of proteins that block blood flow. Based on laboratory animal research, results show anti-tumor activity, and most nutritionists believe that adding shiitake mushrooms to your diet will result in helping fight prostate, breast, and colon cancers. They're rich in several B vitamins and vitamin D, selenium, zinc, and copper; their antioxidant activity is important to keeping cells, especially cardiovascular cells, healthy.

Look for dried shiitake mushroom powder in natural/health food stores and stir a teaspoon into juice or smoothies.

Tomatoes

Red-, orange-, and tangerine-colored tomatoes are high in *lycopene,* one of several antioxidants they contain. One of lycopene's benefits is in boosting bone density and protecting against osteoporosis, especially in women. Fresh tomatoes have also been shown to help lower LDL (bad) cholesterol, and their excellent antioxidants, including lycopene, make them extremely important to heart health. Tomatoes are high in vitamin C and biotin and are a good source of vitamins A, E, and K, potassium, copper, manganese, and fiber.

Add 1 or 2 fresh tomatoes to summer smoothies and juice ingredients. In winter, add one or two canned tomatoes or pure tomato sauce to smoothies.

Astragalus

Astragalus (*Astragalus membranaceus*) is a hardy plant that has been used in traditional Chinese medicine for thousands of years. According to the University of Maryland Medical Center, it may help protect the body from diseases, such as cancer, heart disease, and diabetes. It's an *adaptogen,* meaning that it helps protect the body not only against diseases, but also against mental or emotional stress. In China, it's used in soups and stews and is a favorite herb for the very young and the very old, but everyone can benefit from using it.

The antioxidants along with antibacterial and anti-inflammatory properties in astragalus support your immune system, preventing colds, flu, and upper respiratory infections; protecting the liver and kidneys; lowering cholesterol and blood pressure and protecting the heart; and helping to mitigate diabetes and also the negative effects of chemotherapy.

Look for dried sliced astragalus root and dried root powder in Asian markets or natural/health food stores. Use sliced root in soup stock and broth and add to stews while cooking and remove before serving. Add a ½ teaspoon of the powdered root to smoothies or stir into juice.

Burdock

Burdock (*Arctium lappa*) is a common plant — weed actually — that is now being cultivated for use as a medicinal herb. If you harvest the fresh root, you can use it raw in juices or smoothies because the taste is sweetly nutty. The fresh root may also be cooked and eaten as you would parsnips or carrots.

Its excellent antioxidant, anti-inflammatory, and antibacterial properties give burdock root the ability to protect against colds and flu and other respiratory conditions. Its antibacterial and antifungal sesquiterpene lactones inhibit the growth of bacteria and fungi, which helps prevent infection. Burdock has been used to help protect against some forms of cancer, and because the herb is a powerful immune booster, it may help your body fight off the human immunodeficiency virus (HIV). If you have HIV, its ability to cleanse the bloodstream and lymphatic system of toxins helps your body to prevent the progression of AIDS.

You can find dried burdock root powder in natural/health food stores. Add a ½ teaspoon to smoothies and juice.

Cayenne Pepper

Early studies on cayenne (also referred to as hot chilé) peppers (*Capsicum annuum*) show that they may prevent cancerous lung and liver tumors. Health professionals use their therapeutic properties for easing upset stomach, ulcers, sore throat, coughs, and diarrhea. They also have the ability to break up and move congested mucus, thus helping to speed cold and flu relief.

Cayenne pepper helps the body digest food, and it heats the body, causing it to sweat, which makes it effective as a good detox support and addition to cleansing drinks. High in vitamin A, it also contains vitamin E and B6 as well as iron, phosphorus, copper, and selenium.

Add an ⅛ teaspoon (or to taste) dried cayenne powder to pre-meal digestive juices and smoothies to stimulate the digestive tract.

For an excellent morning cleanse, combine an ⅛ teaspoon (or more to taste) dried cayenne powder, 1 tablespoon liquid honey, and 1 cup hot water and take immediately upon rising.

Echinacea

Echinacea (*Echinacea purpurea*) is a powerful immune booster. It works by activating the body's own immune cells and anti-inflammatory chemicals, which reduce cold and flu symptoms.

Available in tincture and pill form, to be optimized, echinacea must be taken when your body is at high risk of upper respiratory infection (plane travel, work stress, or exposure to people stricken with the cold or flu) or at the first symptoms of infection. It must be taken in sufficient doses and frequently throughout the first 24 hours so that the body can benefit from its stimulating properties.

Take 20 drops of Echinacea tincture six times a day in juices and smoothies made with antioxidant ingredients. Take for four to six days and stop.

Metric Conversion Guide

∙ ∙

*N*ote: The recipes in this book weren't developed or tested using metric measurements. There may be some variation in quality when converting to metric units.

Common Abbreviations

Abbreviation(s)	What It Stands For
cm	Centimeter
C., c.	Cup
G, g	Gram
kg	Kilogram
L, l	Liter
lb.	Pound
mL, ml	Milliliter
oz.	Ounce
pt.	Pint
t., tsp.	Teaspoon
T., Tb., Tbsp.	Tablespoon

Volume

U.S. Units	Canadian Metric	Australian Metric
¼ teaspoon	1 milliliter	1 milliliter
½ teaspoon	2 milliliters	2 milliliters
1 teaspoon	5 milliliters	5 milliliters
1 tablespoon	15 milliliters	20 milliliters

(continued)

Volume *(continued)*

U.S. Units	Canadian Metric	Australian Metric
¼ cup	50 milliliters	60 milliliters
⅓ cup	75 milliliters	80 milliliters
½ cup	125 milliliters	125 milliliters
⅔ cup	150 milliliters	170 milliliters
¾ cup	175 milliliters	190 milliliters
1 cup	250 milliliters	250 milliliters
1 quart	1 liter	1 liter
1½ quarts	1.5 liters	1.5 liters
2 quarts	2 liters	2 liters
2½ quarts	2.5 liters	2.5 liters
3 quarts	3 liters	3 liters
4 quarts (1 gallon)	4 liters	4 liters

Weight

U.S. Units	Canadian Metric	Australian Metric
1 ounce	30 grams	30 grams
2 ounces	55 grams	60 grams
3 ounces	85 grams	90 grams
4 ounces (¼ pound)	115 grams	125 grams
8 ounces (½ pound)	225 grams	225 grams
16 ounces (1 pound)	455 grams	500 grams (½ kilogram)

Length

Inches	Centimeters
0.5	1.5
1	2.5
2	5.0

Inches	*Centimeters*
3	7.5
4	10.0
5	12.5
6	15.0
7	17.5
8	20.5
9	23.0
10	25.5
11	28.0
12	30.5

Temperature (Degrees)	
Fahrenheit	*Celsius*
32	0
212	100
250	120
275	140
300	150
325	160
350	180
375	190
400	200
425	220
450	230
475	240
500	260

Index

• C •

• *G* •

• N •

• *W* •

• Z •

About the Author

Pat Crocker knows about food, herbs, and health from the ground up. She has enjoyed a long career teaching, researching, writing about, growing, and speaking about healthy food and herbs. A home economist (Ryerson University, BAA, 1975), she taught high school immediately upon graduating from the University of Toronto's Ontario Institute for Studies in Education.

After leaving teaching, Pat started a niche food public relations company, Crocker International Communications, Inc., operating in Toronto with food and consumer accounts. She sold the company, moved to a log cabin on the Saugeen River in southern Ontario, and hosted Riversong Herb Walk and Gourmet Lunch programs in the 1990s.

Now an award-winning author and regular writer for food and garden magazines, Pat's articles have appeared in national and international magazines and newspapers. She has been profiled in *Herbs for Health* and the *Toronto Sun;* on Canada's CTV, CBC, and City Television; and on radio stations throughout the United States and Canada. She lectures about food and herb topics throughout the United States and Canada.

The 2011 International Herb Association Professional Award given for outstanding contributions to the herb industry and the 2009 Gertrude H. Foster award from the Herb Society of America for Excellence in Herbal Literature have both honored Pat. Her books, *The Juicing Bible* and *The Vegan Cook's Bible* have won "Best in the World" awards from the International Gourmand Culinary Guild.

Pat's other books include *Kitchen Herbal; Coconut 24/7; Preserving: The Canning and Freezing Guide for All Seasons; The Juicing Bible; The Smoothies Bible; The Vegetarian Cook's Bible; The Vegan Cook's Bible; The Yogurt Bible; 150 Best Tagine Recipes; Flex Appeal and Everyday Flexitarian: Recipes for Vegetarians and Meat Lovers Alike,* both co-authored with Nettie Cronish; *Oregano: 2005 Herb of the Year; Herbs of the Kasbah; Pelegoniums,* co-authored with Joyce Brobst and Caroline Amidon; and *The Healing Herbs Cookbook.*

Pat's lifework embraces food, her spirit is entwined with plants, and she nourishes readers, listeners, and audiences with her knowledge and love of both.

Dedication

This is a book for people who envision a healthy life for themselves and their families. I dedicate it to you, no matter where you are on the path to healthy living.

Author's Acknowledgments

With 18 books under my pen, I have come to understand how to write cookbooks. I've worked with co-authors, editors, copy editors, food editors, designers, recipe testers, and several publishers. And from each, I have learned more about the business of developing, testing, and writing recipes; researching health issues; and the art of writing. Thanks to all the professionals for sharing what they know.

I was delighted to write this book for John Wiley & Sons Canada. Thanks to Anam Ahmed, acquisitions editor, for asking and Tracy Boggier for persevering.

Elizabeth Kuball is amazing. Although we've never met face-to-face, I know that we would have much to discuss if ever we did. Her editing skills have shaped this book from the Table of Contents forward. Chad Sievers was brilliant editing the second edition.

It's nice to know that someone has your back, and with this book, I had three experts on my team: Emily Nolan tested the recipes, Patty Santelli did the nutrition analysis, and Kristina LaRue, RD, was the technical editor. Thanks for your professional work on this book.

After 18 books, my family and friends know the drill. They give me space and time to do the long and solitary job of crafting words for paper. They nurture me when I just want to linger in a garden or on a trail. And they cook and clean. Thank you, each one, especially Shannon and Gary for loving and caring.

Publisher's Acknowledgments

Senior Acquisitions Editor: Tracy Boggier
Project Editor: Chad R. Sievers
Copy Editor: Chad R. Sievers
Technical Editor: Kristina LaRue, RD
Art Coordinator: Alicia B. South
Illustrations: Elizabeth Kurtzman

Production Editor: Siddique Shaik
Cover Photos: ©iStock.com/fcafotodigital